Neurological Development
from Birth to Six Years

Neurological Development from Birth to Six Years

Guide for Examination and Evaluation

Claudine Amiel-Tison, M.D.,

and Julie Gosselin, Ph.D., O.T.

Translated by Carolyn Bastable

THE JOHNS HOPKINS UNIVERSITY PRESS
Baltimore & London

© 1998 Hôpital Sainte-Justine
English translation © 2001 Hôpital Sainte-Justine
All rights reserved. Published 2001
Printed in the United States of America on acid-free paper
9 8 7 6 5 4 3 2 1

The Johns Hopkins University Press
2715 North Charles Street
Baltimore, Maryland 21218-4363
www.press.jhu.edu

Library of Congress Cataloging-in-Publication Data

Amiel-Tison, Claudine.
    [Développement neurologique de la naissance à 6 ans. English]

    Neurological development from birth to six years : guide for examination
and evaluation / Claudine Amiel-Tison and Julie Gosselin ; translated by
Carolyn Bastable.
          p.   cm.
    Includes bibliographical references (p.   ) and index.
    ISBN 0-8018-6564-6 (pbk. : acid-free paper)
    1. Pediatric neurology.   2. Developmental neurobiology.   3. Infants—
Growth.   4. Children—Growth.   5. Neurological examination.
I. Gosselin, Julie.   II. Title.
    RJ488.A454   2001
    618.92'8—dc21   00-009626

A catalog record for this book is available from the British Library.

Contents

Figures

Foreword

No single person has made a greater contribution to the understanding of neonatal neurology than Claudine Amiel-Tison. I am both honored and delighted to write the Foreword to the English edition of this schedule for evaluating neurological development in children from birth to 6 years.

Shortly after she graduated in medicine, Dr. Amiel-Tison decided to specialize in pediatrics. Early on, she was influenced by André Thomas, a specialist in adult neurology, and his assistant, Suzanne Saint-Anne Dargassies. On retiring, André Thomas said he was going to devote the rest of his life to understanding the maturation of the central nervous system. He set up a study of newborns with Julian de Ajuriaguerra, and later with Suzanne Saint-Anne Dargassies. Dr. Thomas's first task was to define the terms *passive tone* and *active tone,* then he set out to devise reproducible methods for measuring them. Claudine Amiel-Tison and her collaborator, Julie Gosselin, use the same definitions and methods in their sophisticated schedule, presented in this book.

Dr. Amiel-Tison was impressed by the findings of her study of cerebral damage in full-term infants in the 1960s, and she published the data in a paper in 1969.[1] She found that if the infant was fully breast or bottle fed by 10 days of age, the outlook was good, no matter how seriously compromised the infant had been at birth; otherwise, one could not be certain of the outcome until the child was past 9 months of age. We still cite that paper today. Dr. Amiel-Tison was determined to devise an assessment for clinicians to use at the cotside that would be reproducible, predictive, and user-friendly.

I first met Dr. Amiel-Tison at a conference in 1972, at which she was speaking on the follow-up of infants presenting with neurological abnormalities in the first days of life. Shortly after, she visited our group in the Department of Paediatrics, University College London Medical School, and demonstrated her techniques. We were so impressed with these techniques that, when we set up a study into the outcome of brain lesions detected by ultrasound in very preterm infants, we incorporated them into our methods.

The assessment schedule has undergone many changes. Dr. Amiel-Tison published the original assessment, for infants from birth to 1 year, in 1976[2] and then in 1978 she began a long and fruitful collaboration with Albert Grenier. Together, they published the first version of the assessment schedule in French in 1980 and a revised version in 1985; the latter was translated into English by Roberta Goldberg.[3-5]

When, in 1979, we began our study in the Department of Paediatrics, University College London Medical School, on the outcome of brain lesions detected by ultrasound in the newborn period in very preterm infants, we used the assessment schedule published by Dr. Amiel-Tison in 1976. Over the following years we modified the schedule, with the help of Dr. Amiel-Tison, to include assessments at 30 months and 4 years of age, and we published our findings on the prediction of neurodevelopmental status at 4 years and 8 years of age from neurodevelopmental status at 1 year of corrected age.[6, 7] Together with Dr. Amiel-Tison, we recently published an abstract on the prediction of school performance at 14 to 15 years of age from neurodevelopmental status at 1 year of corrected age.[8]

Dr. Amiel-Tison had always regretted that the assessment published in 1976 was applicable only up to 1 year of age. She realized that, between us, we had collected a lot of data on 4 year olds, and we combined these with the data collected by Suzanne Saint-Anne Dargassies on 2 year olds to form a single database covering birth to 4 years. We discovered, for example, that in measures of passive muscle tone, the angles changed gradually up to 18 months and little thereafter up to 4 years of age. For the first time, we included a scoring system strictly for research purposes. Shortly after this analysis, we were invited to write an "Experience and Reason" article, published in 1989, which included assessments for children up to 5 years old.[9] And in 1990 we made a video in London (English and French versions) with Dr. Amiel-Tison, demonstrating the methods on children in our ultrasound cohort.[10]

Dr. Amiel-Tison has long been interested in the effect of subtle neurological signs and their role in determining eventual outcome. She was impressed by the paper published by Cecil Drillien,[11] which gave the first description of apparently transient neurological signs. Dr. Drillien had found such signs were associated with poor school performance, and Dr. Amiel-Tison postulated that these subtle neurological signs would predict moderately low IQ and suboptimal school performance —and she was right.[7, 8] We have called the children with this constellation of minor signs "the apparently normal survivors."[12] Dr. Amiel-Tison believes the subtle neurological signs are actually permanent[12] and that examiners can find them if they look for them, at least in adolescents.

Neurological Development from Birth to Six Years is clearly written and beautifully illustrated by Claudine Amiel-Tison and her sister, Annette Tison. The "evaluation grids" in the examination chart are clear and easy to use. This English translation will allow the schedule to be used worldwide; it is a great achievement and I wish it every success.

Ann Stewart, F.R.C.P.
Honorary Senior Lecturer, Department of Paediatrics,
University College London

References

1. Amiel-Tison C. Cerebral damage in full-term newborns: aetiological factors, neonatal status and long term follow-up. *Biol Neonate* 1969;14: 234–250.
2. Amiel-Tison C. A method for neurologic evaluation within the first year of life. *Curr Probl Pediatr* 1976;7(1):1–50.
3. Amiel-Tison C, Grenier A. *Évaluation neurologique du nouveau-né et du nourrisson.* Paris: Masson; 1980.
4. Amiel-Tison C, Grenier A. *La surveillance neurologique au cours de la première année de la vie.* Paris: Masson; 1985.
5. Amiel-Tison C, Grenier A. *Neurological Assessment during the First Year of Life.* Goldberg R, trans. New York: Oxford University Press; 1986.

6. Stewart AL, Costello AM de L, Hamilton PA, Baudin J, Bradford BC, Reynolds EOR. Relation between neurodevelopmental status at one and four years in very preterm infants. *Dev Med Child Neurol* 1989;33:756–765.

7. Roth SC, Baudin J, Pezzani-Goldsmith M, Townsend J, Reynolds EOR, Stewart AL. Relation between neurodevelopmental status of very preterm infants at one and eight years. *Dev Med Child Neurol* 1994;36:1049–1062.

8. Roth S, Baudin J, Townsend J, Rifkin L, Rushe T, Amiel-Tison C, Stewart A. Prediction of extra educational provision at 14–15 years from neurodevelopmental status at one year of corrected age in subjects born before 33 weeks gestation [abstract]. *Pediatr Res* 1999;45:904.

9. Amiel-Tison C, Stewart A. Follow-up studies during the first five years of life: a pervasive assessment of neurological function. *Arch Dis Child* 1989;64:496–502.

10. Amiel-Tison C, Stewart A. *Neuromotor Assessment during the First Five Years of Life* [videotape, English and French versions]. London: UCL Images; 1990. (Distribution: Audiovidéothèque, Hôpital Sainte-Justine, Montréal.)

11. Drillien CM. Abnormal neurologic signs in the first year of life in low birth weight infants: possible prognostic significance. *Dev Med Child Neurol* 1972;14:572–584.

12. Amiel-Tison C, Stewart A. Apparently normal survivors: neuromotor and cognitive function as they grow older. In: Amiel-Tison C, Stewart A, eds. *The Newborn Infant: One Brain for Life*. Paris: Les Éditions INSERM; 1994:227–237.

Acknowledgments

We would like to express special thanks to those people who so generously contributed to the development of this work. We thank Annette Tison for the elegance and precision of her drawings, working from her model, the "balsa-boy," to illustrate each maneuver. We thank Françoise Lebrun for her critical eye in tracking vague descriptions and obscurities, and Bernadette Valpréda for the quality of her technical assistance, making repeated corrections without voicing a single complaint. Madeleine Leduc made the examination chart both pragmatic and aesthetically pleasing: a great-looking chart is much more pleasant to use. Luc Bégin added a professional touch with his meticulous revision of the manuscript. And we are grateful to Sheila Gahagan for her careful reading of the English translation and her much appreciated encouragement, and to Marilee C. Allen for her warm support at all stages, including her skillful assistance with the translation.

Neurological Development
from Birth to Six Years

Chapter 1

Introduction

- A Single Tool Used throughout Infancy and Childhood
- Presentation of Technical Descriptions
- Pathophysiological Basis for Interpretation of Results
- A Summary of Short- and Long-Term Profiles: Deviant Patterns

A Single Tool Used throughout Infancy and Childhood

This book presents a single tool for the neurological examination of children from birth to school age, designed to meet the specific needs of clinicians, researchers, and administrators. Each professional group has different requirements. Perinatologists need to evaluate the technical advances in Neonatal Intensive Care Units based on short- and long-term outcomes of the survivors. Researchers need to thoroughly explore the correlations between risk factors, brain damage, and sequelae. Epidemiologists, in order to identify trends, must be able to compare results from different facilities and from different countries. And public health administrators must be able to evaluate results so as to verify the effectiveness of their health policies.

To meet these various needs, the clinical assessment tool must be both simple and precise. It must be based on a fixed set of observations and maneuvers, and results must be scored according to the child's age, because cerebral maturation, especially during the first year, constantly modifies the results.

It is with these goals in mind that we present here a basic neurological examination that can be used throughout infancy and childhood, while trying to avoid the pitfalls of oversimplification and unnecessary complexity.

We have designed a chart (see "Examination Chart") on which examiners can record the results of each observation or maneuver. Explanations for each maneuver are given in Chapter 3, "Technical Descriptions of Observations and Maneuvers," along with instructions for scoring the results. These maneuvers have been selected based on the results of previous research.[1, 2]

The history behind this neurological development examination began with the method described by André Thomas and Suzanne Saint-Anne Dargassies for newborns,[3] and was further developed with the technique described by Saint-Anne Dargassies for infants during the first years of life.[4] Claudine Amiel-Tison set out to describe the first year of life with the help of a monthly examination chart and a didactic indicator of expected development.[5-7] The summary of results was based on the notion of symptomatic clusterings and deviant profiles. Next,

Amiel-Tison and Ann Stewart extended the method to children 5 years of age in order to conduct neurological follow-ups in a group of children at risk, and they proposed a scoring system.[8] This scoring system, however, was limited to two age groups: 9 to 17 months (an age range characterized by marked physiological hypotonia) and 18 months to 5 years.

This undertaking had a favorable effect in several important areas:

1. Because the technique was simple and easy to reproduce, pediatricians could use the neurological examination for children's first year of life, and whenever the results of repeated examinations were suboptimal during these first months, early intervention could be implemented. This alone represented considerable progress in pediatric practice.

2. The technique allowed a distinction between neurological abnormalities and their functional consequences. The sole use of developmental scales derived from the work of Arnold Gesell does not allow one to distinguish between neurological impairments, which are permanent, and functional consequences, which are age-dependent.

3. With a more precise understanding of moderate and minor abnormalities, it was possible to establish a continuum of cerebral damage, a continuum that had often been disputed because of inadequate methodology.

4. An objective neurological basis enabled examiners to identify children in the first year of life who were at risk of learning disabilities, even though at kindergarten age they showed no apparent signs of dysfunction. This neurological marker represented progress in the analysis of perinatal causes of late dysfunction.[9]

The new neurological development examination presented in this book is the continuation of Amiel-Tison's first endeavor. It allows a single tool to be used for children from birth to 6 years while standardizing examination methods and providing a better presentation and easier interpretation of results. The examination chart itself is presented in the most aesthetic way possible. With this new project, the pragmatism of occupational therapists has played a significant role in simplifying the approach, making it more accessible for daily pediatric practice. Our method offers two possibilities: to confirm neurological optimality early in life despite the perinatal risk factors, or to detect and follow up on a set of neurological signs through infancy and childhood.

Presentation of Technical Descriptions

A technical description of each observation or maneuver is provided in Chapter 3. Typical or atypical results are analyzed according to age and matched with the necessary scoring instructions. The neurological assessment techniques are presented in the same order as they appear in the examination chart. To make these descriptions easier to use, each maneuver also is listed in the index at the end of the book.

The examination norms were derived from the work of Saint-Anne Dargassies on normal development between 0 and 2 years[4] and from the results of studies by Amiel-Tison and Stewart and their colleagues.[10-15] Because of the variations in muscle extensibility at different stages of maturation, we have slightly modified the scoring for muscle extensibility standards. Especially for items related to resistance to slow stretch, variation in muscle extensibility can be due to genetics or lifestyle or both. These variations are neither related to perinatal insult nor pathological. We thought it wise to establish acceptable limits of normalcy based on previous research and the experience of both authors with diverse populations.

This neurological examination is very traditional, except for the evaluation of passive muscle tone, which is more typical of the French school. The reliability of the passive muscle tone evaluation has been tested, and results vary for each maneuver: excellent for the scarf sign, good for both the dorsiflexion and popliteal angles, and poor for the adductors angle.[6] The degree of reproducibility of the maneuvers depends more on the manipulation itself than on visual estimation of the position or angle.

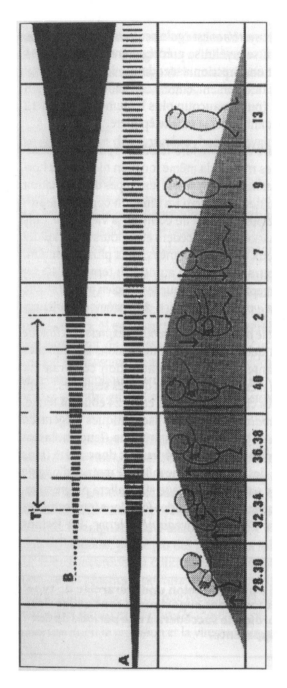

FIG. I. DEVELOPMENT OF UPPER MOTOR FUNCTION CONTROL

Age is indicated in weeks of gestation, then in postnatal months. *A*: the ascending wave of subcorticospinal system maturation; *B*: the descending wave of corticospinal system maturation; *T*: the transitional period from six weeks before to six weeks after full term. The gray area illustrates the waxing and waning pattern of central nervous system control of motor function. (Reprinted with permission from C. Amiel-Tison. *L'infirmité motrice d'origine cérébrale*. Paris: Masson; 1997.)

Pathophysiological Basis for Interpretation of Results

To remain within the framework of a user manual for neurological development assessment techniques, we present here a deliberately simplified pathophysiological approach, which can efficiently guide clinicians in interpreting results for normal development and neuromotor abnormalities.

Interpretation is based on the progressive individualization of two distinct motor control systems: the *subcorticospinal* and *corticospinal systems*. The subcorticospinal system (or *lower system*) originates in the tectum, the reticular formation, and the vestibular nuclei. It therefore issues from the brain stem and is also referred to as the *extrapyramidal system*. The corticospinal system (or *upper system*) originates in the motor and premotor cortex; it is also referred to as the *pyramidal system*.

Each of these systems has a distinct function. The principal role of the mesencephalic, subcorticospinal system (archaic, because it originates in the phylogenetically oldest cerebral structures) is to maintain both erect posture against gravity and flexor tone in the upper limbs. The corticospinal system (which is, phylogenetically speaking, a more recently developed structure that accounts for the gradual encephalization of motor control) is responsible for posture control through inhibitory or excitatory effects on lower structures. It therefore moderates postural hyperextension in the axis and hyperflexion in the upper limbs. In addition to posture, the corticospinal system plays a predominant role in the control of fine motor skills, particularly independent finger movements and rapid, precise, manipulative skills.

These systems also differ in maturation timing (Fig. 1). In the subcorticospinal system, myelination occurs early, between 24 and 34 weeks of gestation, proceeding in a caudocephalic (ascending) direction. In the corticospinal system, myelination begins later, proceeding quickly between 32 weeks of gestation and 2 years of age, then at a considerably slower rate until 12 years, in a cephalocaudal (descending) direction toward the spinal cord.

A knowledge of this maturation schedule helps pediatricians understand normal development. Knowing that the two systems have neither the same function nor the same maturation timetable, clinicians can follow the stages of maturation when evaluating neuromotor function. In fact, archaic-type neuromotor control prevails in fetal life, followed by an "encephalization" phase that continues rapidly throughout the first two years, proceeding more slowly thereafter. The transitional phase from one system to the other (around the full-term period) is of particular interest, because clinicians can monitor development of control of the upper system over the lower system from week to week.

This maturation schedule also helps pediatricians understand the various clinical signs. Since the topography of perinatal ischemic lesions depends on the stage of cerebral maturation at the time of the insult,[2] it is not surprising that sequelae are clearly different in preterm and full-term infants. In the preterm newborn, ischemic lesions occur primarily in the hemispheric white matter (periventricular leukomalacia), altering upper motor control with a severity depending on the extent of the lesions. Cerebral palsy (CP), usually spastic, sets in gradually during the first year of life without significantly affecting intellectual function. In the full-term newborn, asphyxial lesions generally occur in the gray matter (cortex, basal ganglia, and, in the most serious cases, brain stem). Severe mental and sensory deficits are usually associated with CP in these children.

Although admittedly simplified, this description of the maturation schedule provides clinicians with the basic knowledge necessary to conduct neurological examinations within the first years of life and to interpret abnormalities.

NOTE

Cerebral function is organized according to a military-style hierarchy, in which higher neurological functions regulate several lower functions. If higher cortical functions have been destroyed, extreme disorganization is difficult to detect at first and sets in after a variable period of time.

A Summary of Short- and Long-Term Profiles: Deviant Patterns

We believe the most effective approach is to describe typical abnormal profiles for each age so as to help clinicians cluster detected abnormalities. The goal is to encourage the use of step-by-step synthesis rather than computerized data, and this method therefore remains entirely within the problem-solving method. It does not lead to a score, but rather to a pattern of deviancy.

The abnormal sign clusters are presented in tables in Chapter 4, first for each three-month interval then for each six-month interval up to the age of 2 years. The clinician should not accept or dismiss the possibility of CP until a child is at least 2 years old. This helps avoid a prematurely inaccurate diagnosis. Later, between ages 2 and 6 years, a more comprehensive and schematic profile is vital for a child's follow-up and for publishing results. This is why sections are provided in the examination chart for annual profiles that include neuromotor impairments and disabilities, as well as related deficits and non-neurological health problems.

This neurological development assessment tool is primarily intended for long-term follow-up studies of newborns at risk of perinatal cerebral sequelae. Risk of this nature is often already identifiable during pregnancy, at delivery, or in the first few days of life, but in some cases it is abnormal signs during the neonatal examination that reveal this risk, despite the lack of any earlier indicative signs. In cases of extensive damage, clinicians can use ultrasound imaging during the first weeks of life to predict unfavorable development. However, when the results of ultrasound imaging are within normal limits, precise neurological evaluations can prove quite valuable.

NOTE

The clockwork unfolding of neuromotor maturation is such that any delay in gross motor milestones has to be considered atypical.

As far as the pattern of changes is concerned, moderate clinical deviations detected in the first three or four months can completely disappear. They can also change during maturation and develop into moderate, persistent neurological abnormalities, similar to those of CP but milder. Rigorous screening of these moderate deviations is of interest not only to epidemiologists but also to the infant and the infant's family, so that they can benefit from early, on-time intervention for each new problem through early childhood.[1, 2, 16]

This is a minimal, basic examination, intentionally reduced to the essentials. When abnormalities are detected, additional clinical investigations are needed for complete evaluation of the child. A few examples are listed below.

1. If neuromotor deviations are present during the first months of life, the Complementary Neuromotor Examination described by Grenier and colleagues[6, 7, 17, 18] and standardized by Gosselin[19] can be used to refine motor assessment.

2. If CP is detected later within the first year, an in-depth analysis of each factor related to the motor deficit (spasticity, muscle shortening, paralysis, and central disorganization) should be completed to help in defining the most appropriate intervention.

3. If swallowing and feeding problems are present, further assessment should be conducted through specific examination of these functions.

NOTE
Cerebral palsy is defined internationally as a persistent (but not unchanging) disorder of posture and movement caused by a nonprogressive defect or lesion of the immature brain.

NOTE
In the clinical picture of CP, paralysis is underestimated during the first years of life because it cannot yet be evaluated and is masked by spasticity.

---

4. This examination does not cover prelinguistic skills and language development, but the clinician should not omit the assessment of these skills. For the prelinguistic phase and up to 3 years, the Clinical Linguistic Auditory Milestone Scale (CLAMS)[20] can be helpful in defining normalcy or deviation by asking the mother a few questions and by making observations during the pediatric evaluation. If any linguistic abnormalities are observed, more in-depth assessment should be completed by a speech pathologist.

5. If behavioral problems are more conspicuous than the moderate neuromotor abnormalities, pediatricians can use the screening assessment proposed by Baron-Cohen and colleagues[21] for the detection of autism at 18 months. Extending the examination to include functions of play, language, and communication is crucial when psychiatric symptoms are suspected.[22] In more severe cases, a systematic psychiatric assessment should be conducted.

Chapter 2

How to Fill Out the Examination Chart

- Description of the Four Sections of the Examination Chart
- Choosing the Appropriate Column or Line
- Use of Corrected Age up to 2 Years
- Scoring and Recording Results

Description of the Four Sections of the Examination Chart

The chart is designed to record results for ten successive examinations (designated I through X) during the first six years of life. Because cerebral maturation is very rapid during the first year of life, scoring standards change every three months. During the second year, cerebral maturation progresses at a slower rate and the scoring standards change every six months. After the age of 2 years, cerebral maturation is much slower and scoring for this age category does not change, except for acquisition of new motor skills, found under "Motor Development Milestones" in the examination chart.

The examination chart consists of four sections and a profile summary sheet, which includes a classification at 2 years of age and subsequent annual profiles up to 6 years of age. The first section, five pages in length, is general in content and should be completed at each examination. The next three sections (four pages each) are to be used during neurological examinations according to age: 1st to 9th months (examinations I, II, and III); 10th to 24th months (examinations IV, V, and VI); and 3rd to 6th years (examinations VII, VIII, IX, and X).

General Section

This section (section 1, pages 1 to 5) is completed at each examination.

- Page 1 summarizes the series of examinations from 0 to 6 years. Roman numerals I through X correspond to each age category. Columns or lines are chosen according to the child's age at the time of the examination, as indicated by the instructions in Chapter 3. The child's life environment and any subsequent changes in the child's life should also be noted. If the examination is conducted under clearly unfavorable conditions, this should be noted under "Comments."

- Page 2 provides descriptions of changes in head circumference, height, and weight.

- Page 3 enables examiners to record health problems and the morphology of the skull and face.

- Page 4 outlines neurosensory functions, seizures, alertness, attention, and excitability.

- Page 5 summarizes the neuromotor skills generally acquired in the first two years of life (the motor milestones correspond to examinations I through VI).

Three Age-Dependent Neurological Sections

Each of the next three sections is made up of four pages and describes passive tone, motor activity, reflexes, and postural reactions.

- Pages 6 to 9 (section 2) include examinations I, II, and III, conducted between 0 and 9 months of age at three-month intervals.

- Pages 10 to 13 (section 3) include examinations IV, V, and VI, conducted between 10 and 12 months, 13 and 18 months, and 19 and 24 months, respectively.

- Pages 14 to 17 (section 4) include examinations VII, VIII, IX, and X, conducted annually between 2 and 6 years of age.

Summary Profiles at 2 Years (Corrected Age) and up to 6 years

- Page 18 includes a classification for cerebral palsy at 2 years (corrected age) and subsequent annual profiles up to 6 years, summarizing examinations VII through X.

Choosing the Appropriate Column or Line

Roman numerals I through X, which appear at the top of columns or at the left side of lines, correspond to the current month or year. For each examination, examiners choose the column or line that matches the child's age. For example, examiners will use column I from 0 to 3 months, that is, during the child's first, second, and third months. Once the child has begun his or her fourth month, examiners will use column II.

Use of Corrected Age up to 2 Years

For children born before 37 weeks of gestation, the examiner should use the age corrected for degree of prematurity until the child is 2 years old. The corrected age is calculated by subtracting the child's gestational age from 40 weeks and then subtracting this difference from his or her chronological age at the time of testing.

Scoring and Recording Results

Recording the measured value under each heading of the examination chart will ensure that no information is lost.

The examiner circles a score of 0, 1, or 2, according to the information given in the technical descriptions for each maneuver (Chapter 3). The scoring system is as follows:

- A score of 0 indicates a typical result for that age, within the normal range.

- A score of 1 indicates a moderately abnormal result for that age.

- A score of 2 indicates a definitely abnormal result.

For certain items scoring is considered inappropriate, and examiners circle an "X" to indicate examination results (e.g., the plantar reflex on extension during the first year, or the presence of primitive reflexes

> NOTE
> The use of corrected age up to 2 years is sufficient for evaluating neuromotor function, but the use of corrected age should be continued after 2 years of age when evaluating language in extremely preterm children.

during the fourth, fifth, and sixth months). No conclusions should be made regarding the normal or abnormal nature of these results.

A gray shaded area indicates that the item does not have to be tested for that particular age column (e.g., comparison of slow and rapid dorsiflexion angles of the foot during the first three months of life).

Chapter 3

Technical Descriptions of Observations and Maneuvers

- Head Circumference and Growth

- Craniofacial Examination

- Neurosensory Examination

- Observations and Interview

- Motor Development Milestones in the First Two Years

- Passive Muscle Tone

- Motor Activity

- Deep Tendon and Cutaneous Reflexes

- Primitive Reflexes

- Postural Reactions

- Qualitative Abnormalities in Gross Motor Function and Acquired Deformities

Head Circumference and Growth

Head circumference (HC) is obtained by measuring the maximum occipitofrontal circumference of the head. A comparison of measurement values with the norms for children of the same sex and age (e.g., UK Growth Charts)[23] permits statistical definition of a normal range—that is, the range between two standard deviations (SD) above and 2 SD below the average (or between the 2nd and 98th percentiles). Measurements that fall beyond these limits, either too high or too low, constitute abnormal findings. Examiners should record results as follows.

SCORING

- Circle 0 if HC is within the normal range for the child's age and sex, that is, within ±2 SD.

- Circle 2 if HC is higher than 2 SD above the average (macrocephalic) or lower than 2 SD below (microcephalic).

This universal definition of macrocephaly and microcephaly is not entirely adequate because the normal range is very wide and genetic factors play a significant role (see below). Examiners can use the two following methods to refine their interpretation.

Observation of Concordance or Discordance with Other Growth Parameters

The examiner should check whether other growth measurements (height or weight) are concordant or discordant with HC. It is generally accepted that a significant discrepancy between HC and other anthropometric parameters, especially if detrimental to HC, increases the probability of abnormality, even if HC is within the normal range. A difference of 2 SD between HC and other growth parameters can be arbitrarily considered abnormal. In children with hypoxic-ischemic lesions, only a relative decrease in HC with respect to weight or length (not an increase) is worth recording, since it is probably due to cerebral atrophy. In such cases, scoring should be recorded as follows.

- If HC is 2 SD below weight or length, relative microcephaly should be recorded by circling "X."

Head Growth Profile during the First Two Years

Children with HC values that generally follow the same percentile on the growth curve have a greater chance of having normal brain function than children with HC values that either fall below or rise above the initial percentile. In cases of hypoxic-ischemic lesions, a drop in brain growth velocity is usually expected, which may or may not catch up (correct itself) later. Head growth is especially important during the first two years; this is a very active period for development in the cerebral hemispheres. Consequently, scoring should be recorded as follows.

SCORING

- If head growth has been slowing down by at least 1 SD or more and later catches up to the initial curve, examiners should record this information by circling "X" next to "Downward profile with catch up."

- If head growth has been slowing down and then remains on a curve lower than 1 SD from the neonatal value, then, despite being within normal limits, brain growth remains below expected potential. Examiners should record this information by circling "X" next to "Downward profile without catch up."

Development of hydrocephalus is an acute condition; no score is given when HC values indicate that the brain has grown too quickly.

Craniofacial Examination

Ventriculo-peritoneal Shunt

A ventriculo-peritoneal shunt may have been placed as palliative treatment of hydrocephalus. Examiners should indicate the presence of a shunt with an "X," whether or not the shunt is still functioning.

Anterior Fontanel

A rapid increase in brain size during the first year of life is a determining factor in cranial growth. The skull, composed of separate bones at this age, normally undergoes a significant increase in volume made possible by the still-open fontanels and unfused sutures. However, if a deficiency in cerebral growth develops, fontanels may close quickly and cranial sutures may begin to overlap and fuse too early. Consequently, these types of cranial signs are often associated with moderate cerebral atrophy. (Since the size of the anterior fontanel can vary significantly, it is not of clinical interest here. Examiners should be concerned only with its appearance, that is, whether open or closed.)

SCORING

- Circle 0 if anterior fontanel is open.
- Circle 1 if anterior fontanel has closed prematurely between 9 and 12 months.
- Circle 2 if anterior fontanel has closed very prematurely before 9 months.

No score is given in cases of delayed closure of the anterior fontanel.

Cranial Sutures

Examination of each cranial suture is done by palpation. This includes the parietotemporal suture located above the ear (also called the squamous suture because of its beveled-edge appearance) and the frontal, coronal, sagittal, and occipital sutures.

SCORING

- Circle 0 if sutures are edge-to-edge (which is normal) and thus barely palpable.
- Circle 1 if a ridge is detectable, which is due to overlapping of the bones.

1. A ridge is interpreted as a neurological sign during the first months of life only when severe malnutrition and dehydration have been ruled out.

2. No score is given when separated sutures are detected. This finding suggests an acute transient condition that will either correct itself or will require neurosurgery for the treatment of hydrocephalus.

3. A ridge of one or more sutures (especially the squamous suture) can often be detected despite normal HC values. Though subtle, this sign indicates the need for careful long-term follow-up.

Shape of the Skull

Examiners give a score only when there are obvious deformities.

NOTE
Palpation of the skull is an integral part of neurological examinations conducted during the first few years of life; head circumference values alone are not sufficient for detecting growth abnormalities in the cerebral hemispheres.

- Circle 0 if the shape of the skull appears normal.

- Circle 1 if the shape of the skull appears abnormal.

In addition to cerebral atrophy, the most common abnormality found in infants with hypoxic-ischemic lesions is a narrow receding forehead (frontal bone), which makes the arch of the eyebrows seem to protrude abnormally.

Some skull deformities immediately suggest the existence of cerebral malformations. Descriptions of these deformities can be found in neurological textbooks.[24] To help in identifying specific syndromes, a brief description should be recorded on the examination chart.

Shape of the Palate

Lateral palatine ridges disappear during the last three months of gestation owing to fetal tongue movements. This gives the palate its flat appearance, which is normal in the full-term newborn (Fig. 2). When lateral palatine ridges are present, the palate has a high-arched appearance, suggesting weakness or a lack of tongue movements (Fig. 2).

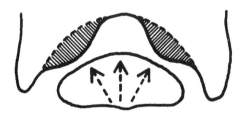

FIG. 2. HIGH-ARCHED PALATE

Lateral palatine ridges usually smooth out with the development of tongue movements during the last months of pregnancy. This creates the normal flat appearance of the palate (dotted line). In cases of abnormal fetal motor activity, lateral palatine ridges are present, giving the palate a high-arched appearance (solid line).

- Circle 0 if the palate has a flat appearance.

- Circle 1 if the palate has a high-arched appearance.

1. When this abnormality is present at full-term birth, it is a sign of a prenatal neurological impairment.

2. This abnormality can also appear later if there are intrapartum or postnatal complications. It is particularly common with brain stem lesions in children with severe cerebral palsy (CP).

3. This is not a pathological sign in very preterm newborns since there has not been sufficient time in utero for the palate to be shaped by sucking movements. In addition, a high-arched palate is often seen in extremely preterm infants after prolonged intubation, presumably due to the presence of the endotracheal tube.

Neurosensory Examination

In this section of the examination chart, only central nerve deficits are analyzed and only the results from clinical assessments are given a score. In cases of uncertain findings or as part of a systematic routine examination, specialized examinations should be conducted to confirm clinical assessments.

NOTE
The fetal tongue is a large, strong, fan-shaped muscle; it contributes to the swallowing of amniotic fluid through rhythmic movements.

Hearing

During the neonatal period, systematic assessments are conducted to check for hearing loss. This is done by observing the newborn's responses to acoustic stimuli such as white noise emitted at a level of 80 to 90 decibels. However, the percentage of false positives and false negatives is quite high.

From 4 months of age, infants are tested with a series of acoustic toys (rattles, clickers, bells, music boxes, etc.).

At approximately 9 months of age, probability of deafness becomes stronger if evidenced by signs observed by the infant's parents: poor vocal sounds; little response when the child's name is whispered or a noise is produced by acoustic toys. When responses are unclear or absent, additional tests are necessary.

SCORING

- Circle 0 if responses are within normal limits.
- Circle 1 if hearing loss is moderate.
- Circle 2 if hearing loss is profound.

Results of additional tests should be fully recorded on the chart, such as audiogram and brain auditory evoked potential (BAEP).

Vision and Ocular Signs

Fix-and-Track. The objects used to elicit "fix-and-track" responses vary with age. During the neonatal period, examiners use a bull's-eye pattern (glossy black and white concentric circles). After the first

---

NOTE
Caution: The babbling sounds of an infant during the first six months are not related to hearing function.

---

month, examiners use the Fantz target (black and white face) or their own faces to attract the infant's attention. At approximately 6 months of age, smaller objects (e.g., pellets) are used.

Results of additional tests should be fully recorded on the chart, such as visual evoked potential (VEP) and electroretinography (ERG).

SCORING

- Circle 0 if fix-and-track responses are present from the first month of life and easily obtained because of a good level of alertness.
- Circle 1 if fix-and-track responses are difficult to obtain and maintain.
- Circle 2 if infant shows no fix-and-track responses.

Nystagmus. Nystagmus, whether horizontal, vertical, or rotatory, must be evaluated (a few jerky eye movements in lateral gaze are not taken into account).

SCORING

- Circle 0 if nystagmus is absent.
- Circle 2 if nystagmus is present.

Eye Movements. Erratic eye movements indicate the absence of fixation.

> NOTE
> Visual impairments make the lives of children with cerebral palsy more difficult. These children should continue to undergo regular follow-up, with repeated eye examinations as they grow.

- Circle 0 if eye movements are synchronous.

- Circle 2 if eye movements are erratic.

Strabismus. Synchronous eye movements are analyzed during the fix-and-track assessment. Strabismus, whether convergent or divergent, unilateral or bilateral, may be observed.

SCORING

- Circle 0 if strabismus is absent.

- Circle 1 if strabismus is present.

> 1. During the first three months of life, strabismus, as long as it is not constant, is considered normal because convergence has not yet been achieved.
>
> 2. If strabismus is constant before 3 months of age, or if it persists after 3 months, an ophthalmologic examination should be conducted.

Sunset Sign. The sunset sign results from a downward deviation of the eyeballs, an indication of a brain stem lesion. The iris is partially covered by the lower eyelid and the sclera is visible above the iris.

SCORING

- Circle 0 if sunset sign is absent.

- Circle 2 if sunset sign is present, whether constant or intermittent.

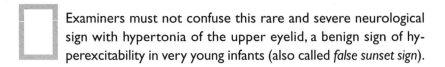

Examiners must not confuse this rare and severe neurological sign with hypertonia of the upper eyelid, a benign sign of hyperexcitability in very young infants (also called *false sunset sign*).

Observations and Interview

Seizures

Types of seizures will not be described here. Whether generalized or focal, the clinical aspects are extremely varied. Parents have difficulty recognizing seizures, particularly in children who are the most seriously affected. Examiners must therefore ask parents simple and straightforward questions about each episode such as: Was the child able to respond to you? Were the child's eyes fixed or turned up? Was the child rigid or limp in your arms? Were the child's limbs shaking? Did the child behave differently the next day?

Seizures that occur when the child has a fever (called *febrile seizures*) do not have the same significance as seizures that have no apparent cause. For this reason, febrile seizures are recorded on the chart but not scored. If the child's temperature is 38°C or higher during the episode, the examiner circles "X."

SCORING

- Circle 0 if seizures are absent.
- Circle 1 for focal or easily controlled seizures.
- Circle 2 for severe, prolonged, and repeated seizures.
- Circle "X" for febrile seizures.

Alertness and Attention

The quality of alertness and attention is determined by a rough estimation based on information from the mother and on observation of the child's behavior during the examination. During the first few months, the response to visual tracking is the most objective method for evaluating alertness and attention. Receptiveness, sociability, smiles, and vocal sounds are other elements of this subjective evaluation. As the child grows, assessment of alertness and attention becomes more qualitative; most often, the child is judged by communication and play during the examination sessions.

SCORING

- Circle 0 if alertness and attention are normal for the child's age.

- Circle 1 for a moderate deficit, as judged by an excessive need for stimulation to obtain sustained participation.

- Circle 2 for a severe deficit, as judged by an almost complete lack of participation despite prolonged encouragement; the mother can confirm whether this lack of alertness is frequently observed or is the result of unusual circumstances.

Hyperexcitability

Hyperexcitability is defined as an excess of excitability. The mother's comments and the examiner's findings during the neurological examination may reveal the following symptoms: insufficient sleep, excessive inconsolable crying, frequent startlings, tremors, and clonic movements.

SCORING

- Circle 0 if signs of hyperexcitability are absent.

- Circle 1 if signs are compatible with normal life.

- Circle 2 if the condition is uncontrollable by usual means.

Motor Development Milestones in the First Two Years

For children with normal cerebral development, a schedule can be established for neuromotor acquisitions, including average age and acceptable time limits. Each of these events or motor development mile-

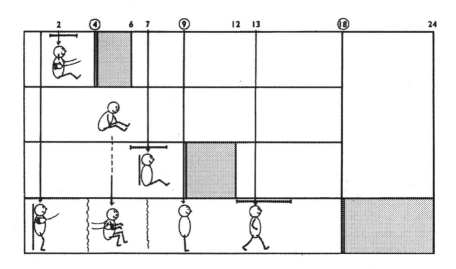

FIG. 3. GROSS MOTOR MILESTONES UNTIL THE AGE OF 2 YEARS

Average age and acceptable time limits are indicated by a double line for the acquisition of each gross motor skill; gray areas indicate a moderate deviation (a score of 1). Note: straightening in the standing position is present at first, then disappears (4 to 6 months), and reappears later when upper motor control has been mastered (8 to 9 months). (Reprinted with permission from C. Amiel-Tison. *L'infirmité motrice d'origine cérébrale*. Paris: Masson; 1997.)

stones reached within a reasonable time frame is given a score of 0 and the exact age of the child is clearly indicated. If a delay is observed, the result is considered moderately pathological and given a score of 1 (gray areas in Figs. 3 and 4). If a more clearly defined delay is observed or the neuromotor acquisition is absent, a score of 2 is recorded (see time limits for each acquisition). Figures 3 and 4 illustrate the motor milestones during the first two years.

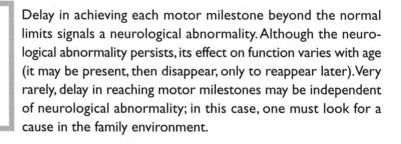

Delay in achieving each motor milestone beyond the normal limits signals a neurological abnormality. Although the neurological abnormality persists, its effect on function varies with age (it may be present, then disappear, only to reappear later). Very rarely, delay in reaching motor milestones may be independent of neurological abnormality; in this case, one must look for a cause in the family environment.

Head Control

To simplify the assessment, the stages of maturation leading to head control are not included in the examination chart. The child's ability to hold up his or her head is the first motor milestone that demonstrates the integrity of higher cortical control. Head control results from balanced contraction of both the flexor and extensor muscles of the neck.

TECHNIQUE

The infant is held in a sitting position. If the head is held steady in the axis of the trunk for at least 15 seconds, head control is present. The average age of acquisition is 2 months.

SCORING

- Circle 0 if head control is present before 4 months of age.

- Circle 1 if head control is acquired during the fifth or sixth month.

- Circle 2 if head control is acquired or absent after 6 months.

> Examiners should stick to the strict definition of head control in the axis of the trunk (see below for possible abnormalities).

Sitting Position

Sitting independently is the result of previous stages (leaning forward on arms, as at 5 months, then without arm support). Independent sitting occurs when the child sits alone for 15 seconds or more without using his or her arms to maintain the posture. The average age of acquisition is 7 months.

- Circle 0 if independent sitting is acquired before 9 months of age.

- Circle 1 if sitting is acquired between the 10th and 12th months.

- Circle 2 if sitting is acquired or absent after 12 months.

Walking Independently

Independent walking occurs when the child can take at least three steps unaided. The average age of acquisition is 13 months.

SCORING

- Circle 0 if independent walking is acquired before 18 months of age.

- Circle 1 if walking is acquired between the 19th and 24th months.

- Circle 2 if walking is acquired or absent after 2 years.

> To a certain extent, falling, or walking with legs wide apart or on tiptoes, is normal until the age of 2 years. These observations are therefore not given a score until that age.

Putting a Cube into a Cup (by Imitation)

The voluntary release of a 2.5 cm cube into a cup with a 10 to 12 cm opening is associated with the gradual disappearance of the grasping reflex.

TECHNIQUE

With the child seated, the examiner places a 2.5 cm cube and a cup in front of the child. The examiner then demonstrates the activity. The child drops the cube into the cup; the wrist should be slightly extended and the child should not lean on the cup for support.

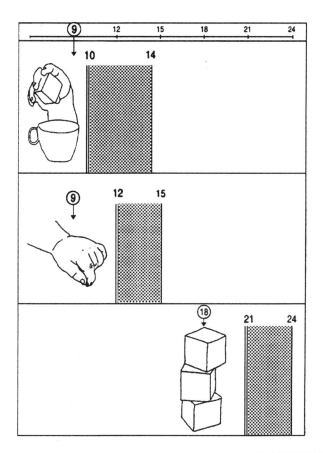

FIG. 4. FINE MOTOR MILESTONES UNTIL THE AGE OF 2 YEARS

The arrows indicate the average age of acquisition, the double lines indicate the acceptable age limit, and the gray areas indicate a moderate delay for the following three fine motor skills: putting a cube in a cup (by imitation), grasping a pellet (thumb-index pinch), and building a three-cube tower (by imitation). (Reprinted with permission from C. Amiel-Tison. *Neurologie périnatale*. Paris: Masson; 1999.)

SCORING

- Circle 0 if putting a cube in a cup is acquired before 10 months
- Circle 1 if this activity is acquired between the 11th and 14th months.
- Circle 2 if this activity is acquired or absent after 14 months.

Grasping a Pellet

Picking up a pellet with the thumb-index pinch requires proper functioning of the corticospinal system. This pinching motion implies dissociation of finger movements and opposition of the thumb.

TECHNIQUE

With the child seated, the examiner places a small 0.5 cm object (such as a raisin) on the table in front of the child. The child grasps the object using thumb-index finger opposition. Slight flexion of the thumb is observed at the metacarpophalangeal joint, and more pronounced flexion is observed at the interphalangeal joint. The child should use the terminal or subterminal surfaces of the thumb and index finger to grasp the object.

SCORING

- Circle 0 if grasping a pellet is acquired before 12 months.
- Circle 1 if this activity is acquired between the 13th and 15th months.
- Circle 2 if this activity is acquired or absent after 15 months.

Building a Three-Cube Tower (by Imitation)

Building a tower using cubes requires good visual motor skills and adequate postural control.

TECHNIQUE

The child is seated at a table adjusted to his or her size; five 2.5 cm cubes are placed on the table in front of the child. The examiner demonstrates the activity once. The child should stack at least three cubes.

- Circle 0 if building a tower is acquired before 21 months.

- Circle 1 if this activity is acquired between the 22nd and 24th months.

- Circle 2 if this activity is acquired or absent after 2 years.

Passive Muscle Tone

Definition: Resistance to Slow Stretching

Examiners use slow passive movements to evaluate muscle tone at rest. In adult neurology, *passive tone* refers to muscle resistance (apart from the effects of gravity or an articular disease) that the clinician notes when moving a joint at rest. By using their own proprioceptive experience, examiners can determine what is too much or too little resistance to motion. Even without the measurement of precise angles, the term *hypertonia* is used when the resistance felt is too strong, and the term *hypotonia* when the resistance felt is too weak.

It is essential to evaluate the range of passive movement during early childhood because of the spectacular changes in tone that occur with maturation (see below). Consequently, the terms *hypertonia* and *hypotonia* imply that the range of passive movement is either too limited or too wide for age standards.

Muscle tone at rest is easy to evaluate in older children and adults, but more difficult to assess in newborns and very young children. Examiners must be aware of the maturational phenomena that affect passive tone during early childhood. These physiological changes, which occur very rapidly at first and more slowly later, indicate the need for an age-dependent scoring system (see below).

> NOTE
> In assessing passive muscle tone, examiners must keep one eye on the angle they are estimating and the other eye on the infant's face, so they can stop the maneuver if the infant grimaces.

The results of each maneuver are expressed as the angle between two segments of a limb (e.g., the popliteal angle), or position in relation to an anatomical landmark (e.g., the elbow in relation to the midline for the scarf sign), or as the amount of curvature (e.g., of the trunk).

Examiners must do the following:

1. Obtain a state of quiet alertness favorable to the child's relaxation.

2. Ensure that the child's head is in the midline in order to avoid eliciting the asymmetric tonic neck reflex.

3. Control the force applied, and stop stretching when the child's discomfort becomes noticeable.

Maturation Profile of Passive Tone in the Limbs from 0 to 6 Years

The development of passive tone in the limbs is illustrated in Figure 5. At first, the stages of maturation are rapid and spectacular. As discussed earlier, at 40 weeks term (or 40 weeks of corrected age in preterm infants), physiological hypertonia of flexor muscles in all four limbs is very strong and under subcorticospinal control. Hence, stretching is very limited (first gray area, labeled "T," in Fig. 5).

During the following months, the descending wave of muscular relaxation (cephalocaudal) is one indication that the upper neuromotor corticospinal system is taking control over the subcorticospinal system. This progression results in physiological hypotonia (second gray

NOTE
Cerebral maturation, a central nervous system phenomenon that determines the descending wave of relaxation, is not significantly affected by the lifestyle of the child.

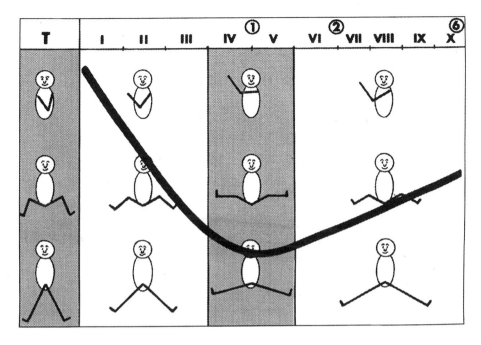

FIG. 5. MATURATION OF PASSIVE TONE IN THE LIMBS FROM
0 TO 6 YEARS

This progression is illustrated by three maneuvers (scarf sign, popliteal angle, and adductors angle), starting with physiological hypertonia, which is characteristic of the full-term infant (gray area, *T*). In nine months, the rapid maturation of the corticospinal system leads to physiological hypotonia (gray area at approximately 1 year of age). After 2 years, resistance to passive manipulation increases with maturation of the musculo-ligamentous system. The Roman numerals refer to the number of the examination; the Arabic numerals refer to the age of the child in years. *T* indicates term (40 weeks gestation).

area, between 9 and 18 months, in Fig. 5). This hypotonia can vary in intensity: there may be a complete lack of resistance to stretching. The age of onset can also vary, usually from 6 to 9 months. This hypotonia may persist until the age of 18 months. Thus the sequence from extreme hypertonia to extreme hypotonia, extending over a period of approximately nine months, is linked to cerebral maturation.

Later, between 2 and 6 years of age and up, there is a very slow, progressive increase in resistance to passive stretching. This phenomenon depends on extracerebral factors. It is linked to the development of muscle mass and the strengthening of articular ligaments and, for this reason, is fairly dependent on the physical activity of the child. A very physically active child will have a musculo-ligamentous system that is more resistant to passive stretching.

In order to include passive tone assessment in the neurological examination of infants and young children, the examiner must do the following:

1. Modify the normal reference values at each three-month interval over the first nine months of life, and at less frequent intervals thereafter.

2. Broaden the definition of normalcy (which is indicated by a score of 0) so that individual, familial, and ethnic variations are taken into account.

3. Keep in mind that a complete lack of resistance to stretching is normal between 9 and 18 months and thus is not given a score.

4. Know how to recognize the abnormality referred to as *benign congenital hypotonia,* in which resistance to stretching is very weak from the first few months of life and remains that way. The family's medical history will reveal hyperextensibility in the ascendants or siblings and will confirm the absence of neurological or muscular disorders, thus denoting an isolated characteristic.

NOTE
Independent walking is acquired during the period of physiological hypotonia. Subsequent maturation of the body (muscles and joints) is variable and depends on the child's physical activity. The progressive increase in resistance to passive stretching is therefore a peripheral phenomenon (due to changes in the musculoskeletal system).

Rapid Stretching and Stretch Reflex Examination: Definition of Spasticity

Like the slow stretching described above, rapid stretching is used to identify a deficit in upper motor control. When the entire neuromotor and muscular system is intact, passive rapid stretching of one segment of a limb should not cause an increase in resistance. The range of motion is comparable to that obtained with slow manipulation. When control is altered, the response to rapid manipulation will change; this is referred to as *spasticity*. Two abnormal responses enable examiners to differentiate between two degrees of severity: the first response (*phasic*) is brisk and of short duration; the second (*tonic*) is more marked and protracted (see below).

Without providing an extensive pathophysiological explanation of spasticity, we can summarize it as follows: lack of upper control of the *myotatic reflex* constitutes the main abnormality, causing *spasticity, hyperreflexia,* and *clonus* (i.e., rhythmic movements of a segment of a limb, set off by a rapid stretching). The intensity of these three signs is usually similar, but small, unexplained variations can be observed. Spasticity is prevalent in the flexor muscles of the upper limbs and in the antigravity extensor muscles of the lower limbs. The presence of all three signs suggests a lesion in either the corticospinal system or the motor cortical areas.

Adductors Angle

TECHNIQUE

With the child supine, the examiner extends the child's legs and gently spreads them as far apart as possible. The angle formed by the two

> NOTE
> During rapid stretching, muscles become stiff unless higher cortical control constantly modulates the action of spinal stretch reflexes.

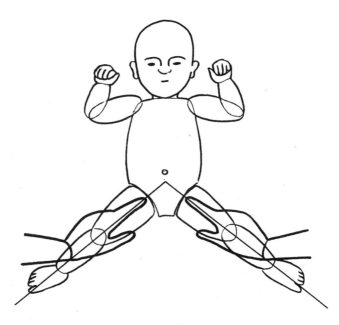

FIG. 6. ADDUCTORS ANGLE

By placing their index fingers parallel to the femoral diaphysis, examiners can easily evaluate the maximum width of the adductors angle (approximately 100° in this diagram).

legs is the *adductors angle*. The extensibility of the left and right adductor muscles (evaluated simultaneously) is measured by the degree of this slow angle (Fig. 6).

PATTERN OF CHANGES

The adductors angle increases progressively over the first nine months. At 2 months of age, it is 40° to 80°; at 9 months, 100° to 140° or more, with the lower limbs offering very little resistance. Between 9 and 18 months, the age of physiological hypotonia, the angle can be limitless. Over the following years, the adductors angle slowly decreases until it reaches average adult measurements.

SCORING

Scoring is age-dependent. (See the examination chart to record a score of 0, 1, or 2.) Adductors angles that fall below age-standard measurements help examiners identify abnormal hypertonia of the adductor muscles.

A complete lack of resistance between 9 and 18 months should be recorded with an "X." If it is detected before 9 months or after 18 months, examiners should record a score of 2.

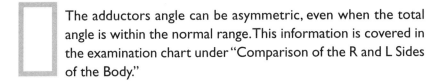

The adductors angle can be asymmetric, even when the total angle is within the normal range. This information is covered in the examination chart under "Comparison of the R and L Sides of the Body."

Popliteal Angle

TECHNIQUE

While keeping the child's pelvis on the table, the examiner laterally flexes both of the child's thighs at the pelvis to each side of the abdomen. With the thighs held in this position, the legs are extended as much as possible. The angle formed by the legs and the thighs is the *popliteal angle*. Both the left and right angles are evaluated at the same time. The measurement of this angle indicates the extensibility of the hamstring muscles (Fig. 7).

PATTERN OF CHANGES

The popliteal angle gradually increases over the first nine months. At 2 months of age it is approximately 90°; at 9 months, 120° to 150°. It can be limitless between 9 and 18 months (the age of physiological hypotonia). The popliteal angle slowly decreases over the following years until it reaches average adult values.

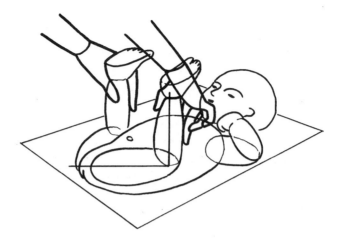

FIG. 7. POPLITEAL ANGLE

With the child's knees held on each side of the abdomen, the examiner extends both of the child's legs as far as possible. The examiner visually evaluates the angle formed between the thigh and the leg (both left and right angles are 90° in this diagram).

SCORING

Scoring is age-dependent. (See the examination chart to record a score of 0, 1, or 2.) Popliteal angles that fall below age-standard measurements help examiners identify abnormal hypertonia of the hamstring muscles. A complete lack of resistance is recorded with an "X" between 9 and 18 months, because the existence of physiological hypotonia is often quite marked; it should be given a score of 2 before 9 months and after 18 months.

Dorsiflexion Angle of the Foot: Slow Maneuver

The dorsiflexion angle as measured by the slow maneuver is also called the *slow angle*. It enables examiners to measure resistance of the resting triceps surae to slow stretching (gray area in Fig. 8).

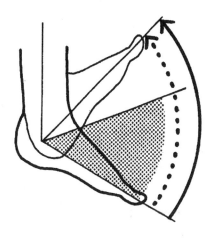

FIG. 8. DORSIFLEXION OF THE FOOT:
NORMAL RESPONSE
Dorsiflexion of the foot is first performed
slowly (dotted line), then rapidly (solid line).
The angles obtained by both manipulations
should be identical and within the normal
range (white area, 80° or less).

TECHNIQUE

The examiner flexes the child's foot toward the leg by slowly pressing
the plantar surface. The angle formed by the longitudinal axes of the
foot and the leg is the *dorsiflexion angle*. This maneuver is performed
on each foot in turn, with the examiner's hand placed on the knee to
keep the leg straight. (This slow angle measures the extensibility of the
triceps surae with the knee extended in order to include the gastroc-
nemius.) The slow angle is the smallest angle obtained by applying
light pressure. When the child is older, the whole foot, including the
heel, is placed in the palm of the examiner's hand to obtain the maximum stretching of the triceps surae.

PATTERN OF CHANGES

Development in the first few months: The starting point varies according to gestational age at birth. The dorsiflexion angle of the foot
is close to 0° in the full-term infant, because the in utero pressure during the last weeks of pregnancy gradually decreases this angle. In the
preterm infant who has reached the age of 40 weeks, the angle remains
wide, as it was at birth (e.g., 40° to 50° at 28 weeks). Later, during the
first few months, the 0° dorsiflexion angle of the full-term infant gradually increases to match the angle of the preterm infant. This is why
this maneuver is performed only after the fourth month, and only an-

gles above the normal upper limit are taken into account (more than 80°; gray area in Fig. 8).

Later development: If permanent dystonia is associated with spasticity detected in the triceps surae (see below), a permanent equine deformity of the foot may result, leading to the shortening of both the muscle and the tendon, thus making the slow angle excessively wide.

SCORING

- Circle 0 if the dorsiflexion angle is equal to or less than 80°.
- Circle 1 if the angle is between 90° and 100°.
- Circle 2 if the angle is equal to or greater than 110°.

> 1. A moderate muscle shortening (90° to 100°) is compatible with normal gait, because only a limited amount of flexion and extension is needed.
>
> 2. A 90° angle is common in very physically active children between 2 and 6 years of age, and this should not be considered "neurological" as long as it is an isolated finding.

Dorsiflexion Angle of the Foot: Rapid Maneuver

The dorsiflexion angle as measured by the rapid maneuver is also called the *rapid angle*. It enables examiners to evaluate the spasticity of the triceps surae.

TECHNIQUE

The same dorsiflexion movement is used as in the slow maneuver, but done more rapidly. The repetition of the manipulation often makes an abnormal response more obvious.

- Circle 0 if the dorsiflexion angle obtained with rapid stretching of the triceps surae is identical to the angle obtained with the slow maneuver (Fig. 8).

- Circle 1 if a sudden yet brief contraction is noted during the rapid maneuver. The resistance quickly dissipates, allowing the foot to attain the position obtained by the slow maneuver. (A few clonic movements often occur with increased resistance.) This response to rapid manipulation is called *phasic* (Fig. 9).

- Circle 2 if the resistance is strong and sustained, if it almost immediately prevents rapid manipulation, and if the movement can only be completed slowly. In this case, the abnormal response to rapid manipulation is called *tonic*. This is the *stretch reflex*, characteristic of the spastic muscle (Fig. 10).

1. The combination of spasticity and shortening of the triceps surae is typical of spastic diplegia (Little's disease). Muscle shortening is secondary to permanent dystonia and often associated with spasticity (which is speed-dependent). Permanent dystonia of the triceps surae causes a permanent equine deformity of the foot and therefore pulls the triceps surae insertions closer together.

2. For scoring purposes, rapid manipulation is systematically tested only in the triceps surae since moderate spasticity is always distal: if moderate spasticity is absent in the triceps surae, it will also be absent in the other muscles. However, if the stretch reflex is present in the triceps surae, the examination should be extended to include the other muscle groups in the lower limbs in order to analyze spasticity muscle by muscle.

FIG. 9. DORSIFLEXION OF THE FOOT: PHASIC STRETCH

The slow angle (dotted line) is within the normal range (80° or less). The rapid angle (solid line) is identical, but a short stop will be felt with or without clonus shortly after starting the maneuver. When this contraction relaxes, the rapid maneuver can be completed to the same extent as the slow maneuver.

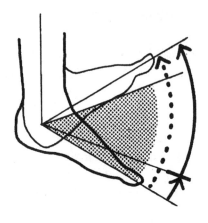

FIG. 10. DORSIFLEXION OF THE FOOT: TONIC STRETCH

The slow angle (full dotted line) is indicated in the gray area (greater than 80°) and suggests a shortening of the triceps surae. The rapid maneuver (lower solid line) is prevented by a very strong contraction of the triceps surae, and dorsiflexion can be continued only slowly (upper dotted line).

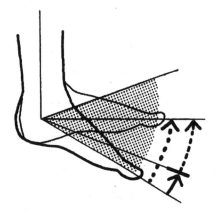

Candlestick Posture

Shortening of the trapezius can be due to prolonged abnormal postures in intensive care units. It is also maintained by almost exclusive use of the ventral and dorsal decubitus positions without particular attention being paid to the upper extremities. Muscular shortening is caused by the medial and external insertions (clavicle, acromion, and the upper ridge of the scapula) being closer to one another. When the child is observed from behind in a sitting or dorsal decubitus position, the arms are seen to be externally rotated and the forearms flexed in such a way that the upper limbs form a two-armed candlestick. Examiners should indicate the presence of this posture by circling "X."

SCORING

- Circle 0 if the candlestick posture is absent.

- Circle "X" if the candlestick posture is present.

1. The candlestick posture (shoulder girdle retraction) is often so marked that it creates a deep crease in the posterior aspect of the arm below the deltoid insertion, resembling a deep gash made by an axe.

2. This posture is abnormal because it results in inactivity of the upper limbs during the critical phase of development when the hands normally join at the midline to manipulate objects.

3. If this posture has been allowed to develop, it can be corrected with physical therapy and by placing the child in appropriate positions during sleep. The candlestick posture is not due to a central neurological disorder, but it should be noted because it prevents a proper neurological examination and impedes the development of manipulative skills.

Hand and Finger Movements

The posture and spontaneous movements of the fingers can be observed from the first neurological examination (Fig. 11).

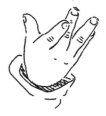 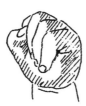 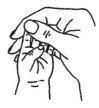

FIG. 11. HAND AND FINGER MOVEMENTS AND POSTURES
Shown from left to right: fine finger movements; closed hand, but can be opened easily; adducted thumb held inside tight fist.

- Circle 0 if an open hand and fine finger movements are observed; this activity is normal when the infant is awake.

- Circle 1 if the hands are constantly closed with no visible finger movements at examination I, conducted between the first and third months, even if the fingers can be spread apart easily.

- Circle 2 if the hands are constantly closed from examination II (fourth to sixth months) onward; and circle 2 at any age if no movement of the thumb is observed and if it remains permanently adducted inside a fisted hand.

1. Abduction of the thumb is a pyramidal function, and inactivity of the thumb is a sign of problems with higher cortical control. When the examiner opens the infant's hand, this posture with the thumb flexed over the palm (shown in Fig. 11) is called *adducted* or *cortical thumb*.

2. Prolonged inactivity results in atrophy (or underdevelopment) of the thenar eminence and in musculo-ligamentous contracture. This must be treated.

3. When thumb adduction is observed from birth, it is highly indicative of a prenatal cerebral lesion. The greater the contracture and atrophy, the older is the lesion.

NOTE
The speed of independent finger movements develops over the first years with the maturation of upper motor control. An intact corticospinal tract is necessary to play the piano.

Scarf Sign Maneuver

This maneuver evaluates the extensibility of the trapezius, the abductors, and the external rotators of the shoulder (the neck is maintained while the acromial insertion of the trapezius is moved).

TECHNIQUE

For infants in the first few months of life, this maneuver is performed as follows. With his or her elbow resting on the examination table, the examiner supports the head and neck of the infant in a semi-supine position with one hand. One of the infant's hands is taken and the arm is pulled across to the opposite shoulder as far as possible. The examiner then observes the position of the elbow in relation to the midline. Later, when the infant can sit independently, the maneuver can be performed with the child in the sitting position, with the observer either behind or in front of the child. At any age, the infant's head must be kept in the midline.

RESULTS

To help examiners with their observations, three elbow positions are illustrated in Figure 12.

- Position 1: elbow does not reach the midline

- Position 2: elbow passes the midline

- Position 3: elbow reaches very far across with little resistance

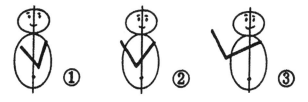

FIG. 12. SCARF SIGN

Position 1: the elbow does not reach the midline; position 2: the elbow passes the midline; position 3: the elbow reaches well past the midline.

If the examiner feels no resistance (NR), this is also noted on the examination chart.

SCORING

Scoring is age-dependent. (See the examination chart to record a score of 0, 1, or 2.) At term, resistance to stretching is very strong and then gradually dissipates. At 2 months, the elbow almost reaches the midline (this is the first indication of the descending wave of relaxation when upper control is intact). At or before 9 months, there is little or no resistance and the arm can be wrapped around the neck. Examiners should give a score for complete lack of resistance only before 9 months or after 18 months of age, not for any age in between, because hypotonia is physiological at this stage of development (9 to 18 months).

Comparison of the Right and Left Sides of the Body: Asymmetry within the Normal Range

As explained above, definition of a wide normal range of passive tone in the limbs is necessary because of individual variations. Asymmetric findings noted during the examination will become evident when comparing the scores of the left and right sides of the body. The examiner should note the following points, however.

1. Asymmetry can be present even when all values (both left and right) have been given a score of 0. This asymmetry represents an abnormality in itself, which is clearly visible and significant within the normal range. It is easier to detect a moderate abnormality when it is unilaterally predominant.

2. Asymmetry can be an important orientation marker for a particular type of cerebral lesion, and therefore the examiner may use information as a diagnostic clue.

- Circle 0 if asymmetry is absent or cannot be categorized.
- Circle 1 if one side (left or right) is more tonic than the other.

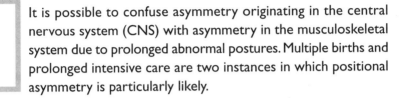

It is possible to confuse asymmetry originating in the central nervous system (CNS) with asymmetry in the musculoskeletal system due to prolonged abnormal postures. Multiple births and prolonged intensive care are two instances in which positional asymmetry is particularly likely.

Passive Extension of the Body Axis (Dorsal Curvature)

Slow dorsal extension of the trunk evaluates the extensibility of the anterior axial muscles (all the prerachidian and abdominal muscles).

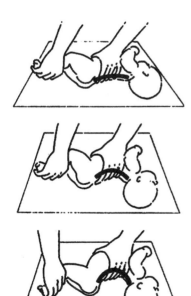

FIG. 13. DORSAL EXTENSION OF THE BODY AXIS
This is evaluated with the child in the lateral decubitus position, with one of the examiner's hands maintaining the lumbar region. Dorsal extension can be absent or minimal (above), moderate (middle), or excessive (below).

With the infant lying on his or her side, the examiner maintains the lumbar region with one hand and pulls the lower limbs backward with the other hand (Fig. 13).

- Circle 0 if dorsal curvature is absent, minimal, or moderate.

- Circle 2 if dorsal curvature is excessive, resulting in arching (also called *opisthotonos*).

Passive Flexion of the Body Axis (Ventral Curvature)

Slow ventral flexion of the trunk evaluates the extensibility of the posterior axial muscles (trapezius and all the paravertebral extensor muscles).

With the infant lying on his or her back, the examiner grasps both the legs and pelvis and pushes them toward the head to test the maximum curvature of the spine (Fig. 14).

- Circle 0 if ventral curvature is moderate but easy to obtain.

- Circle 1 if ventral curvature is absent or minimal.

- Circle 2 if ventral curvature is unlimited, indicating extreme hypotonia.

Comparison of Dorsal and Ventral Curvatures of the Body Axis

A precise definition of the degree of passive flexion and extension of the trunk is impossible. Curvature is evaluated visually, not measured;

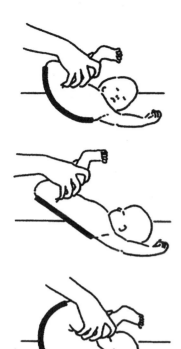

FIG. 14. VENTRAL FLEXION OF THE BODY AXIS

This is evaluated with the child in the dorsal decubitus position. Ventral flexion can be moderate (above), absent or minimal (middle), or unlimited (below).

resistance to passive manipulation is felt through the examiner's hands, not measured. Flexion and extension vary with age, and both values are greater during the period of physiological hypotonia. They also vary with articular and individual factors, as well as poor tolerance for manipulation when the child is in the supine position. It is by comparing both curvatures that examiners arrive at the best interpretation of passive tone of the axis and its deviations. Comparative scoring at any age should be as follows.

SCORING

- Circle 0 if flexion is greater than or equal to extension—that is, there is a certain degree of anterior curvature and little or no dorsal extension. (Flexion and extension are given a score of 0.)

- Circle 1 if flexion is more limited than extension. (Flexion is scored 1 because it is minimal or absent, and extension is scored 0 or 2.)

This situation indicates a lack of upper control of the antigravity muscles.

- Circle 2 if both curvatures are unlimited. (Both are scored 2.) Comparing the scores of the two maneuvers offers no benefit, and findings are interpreted as extreme axial hypotonia (sometimes called rag doll).

Diffuse Rigidity

Rigidity cannot be evaluated in the same way as hypotonia or hypertonia—that is, by measuring muscular extensibility (angles or curvatures). Rigidity is detected as an abnormal sensation during passive manipulation. Slow manipulation gives the examiner a feeling of increased resistance over the whole movement, such as the resistance felt when trying to bend a lead pipe. The detected resistance includes both the agonistic and antagonistic muscles involved in the joint being manipulated.

SCORING

- Circle 0 if rigidity is absent.
- Circle 2 if rigidity is present.

NOTE

Passive tone of the axis is permanently affected in children who lack higher cortical control. If the cerebral lesion is minor, the imbalance in the flexor and extensor muscles is latent and becomes apparent only when the curvatures of the trunk are compared.

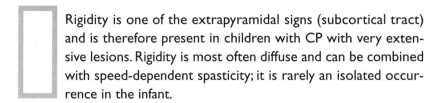

Rigidity is one of the extrapyramidal signs (subcortical tract) and is therefore present in children with CP with very extensive lesions. Rigidity is most often diffuse and can be combined with speed-dependent spasticity; it is rarely an isolated occurrence in the infant.

Motor Activity

Facial Expression

Observation of facial mimicking is part of the neurological examination. Facial expressions are normally greatly diversified and contribute to showing pleasure, pain, and various discomforts.

SCORING

- Circle 0 if facial expressions appear normal, symmetric, and varied.

- Circle 1 if the infant does not show much facial expression, which indicates insufficient facial motility.

Drooling

Constant drooling is a sign similar to facial expression, but it is too insignificant before the age of 1 year to be recorded as abnormal.

SCORING

- Circle 0 if drooling is absent during the first year.

- Circle 1 if drooling is present during the second year.

- Circle 2 if drooling persists significantly after 2 years of age. If this occurs, it is one of a series of severe signs.

- Circle "X" if drooling is present during the first year.

Facial Paralysis

Unilateral or bilateral facial paralysis is scored, and the affected side is indicated.

SCORING

- Circle 0 if facial paralysis is absent.
- Circle 2 if facial paralysis is present.

Fasciculation of the Tongue

Fascicular movements of the tongue are abnormal if they occur at rest and on the sides of the tongue. This is an indication of a lesion in the nucleus of the 12th cranial nerve.

SCORING

- Circle 0 if fascicular tongue movements are absent.
- Circle 2 if fascicular tongue movements are present.

Fascicular movements observed only during crying or only in the central part of the tongue are insignificant and are not given a score.

NOTE

A common misdiagnosis must be noted here. Congenital hypoplasia of the *depressor anguli oris* muscle (autosomal dominant), resulting in a deformation of the mouth, is visible only when the child cries and is not to be confused with facial paralysis.

Spontaneous Limb Movements

Spontaneous limb movements are observed in the supine position during the first few months of life. Later, all gestures are observed. It is difficult to quantify spontaneous motor activity precisely, but a global estimation can be scored.

SCORING

- Circle 0 if limb movements are smooth and varied at all ages.

- Circle 1 if limb movements are insufficient, uncoordinated, or stereotypical.

- Circle 2 if limb movements are barely present or very uncoordinated.

Involuntary Movements

Involuntary movements may appear or increase during the second year. They can be described as rapid, involuntary movements that affect voluntary movements (as in chorea) or as slow, writhing, involuntary movements that interfere with resting postures (as in athetosis). Involuntary movements are an indication of extensive lesions in the extrapyramidal system and hence are often associated with diffuse rigidity. Stereotypical hand movements are very specific to Rett syndrome.

SCORING

- Circle 0 if involuntary movements are absent.

- Circle 2 if involuntary movements are present, and describe the type.

Dystonia

Relatively constant abnormal posture, known as *dystonia,* is due to contractions of the antagonistic muscles, caused by a lack of higher cortical control. Dystonia causes the trunk, the neck, or part of a limb to remain fixed in an extreme position, resulting in a major functional problem.

SCORING

- Circle 0 if dystonia is absent.
- Circle 2 if dystonia is present.

Deep Tendon and Cutaneous Reflexes

Deep Tendon Reflexes

A rough quantitative system has been designed to permit consistency between examiners. In fact, detecting left/right asymmetry is more useful than precisely quantifying the response itself. As far as possible, deep tendon reflexes are tested when the infant is calm and relaxed. Only bicipital and patellar reflexes are scored.

SCORING

- Circle 0 if the deep tendon reflex consists of a few movements with average amplitude.
- Circle 1 if this reflex is very strong.
- Circle 2 if this reflex is accompanied by significant clonus and/or extends to other muscle groups or if there is no response during favorable examination conditions.

NOTE

The terms *spasticity* (speed-dependent) and *dystonia* (abnormal posture) are borrowed from adult neurology and they do not perfectly apply to the clinical description of CP. Central disorganization of neuromotor function is specific to lesions inflicted on a developing brain.

Plantar (Cutaneous) Reflex

The results of plantar reflexes cannot be interpreted during the first year. Results of normal flexion of the big toe after cutaneous stimulation of the outer edge of the foot are inconsistent. If stimulation is too strong, it elicits an extensor reflex, considered meaningless at this age. Because standardization of the stimulation does not seem to be possible, the extensor reflex is not scored until the age of 1 and is indicated with an "X" for younger children.

SCORING

- Circle 0 if flexion of the big toe is observed.

- Circle 2 if extension of the big toe is observed in children over 1 year of age (Babinski sign).

- Circle "X" if extension of the big toe is observed during the first year.

Primitive Reflexes

Primitive reflexes are indicators of subcortical cerebral functioning. The presence of primitive reflexes is physiological during the first months of life, indicating the absence of CNS depression and an intact brain stem. Testing a few of these reflexes will suffice; it is not necessary to check them all. After the first few months, when cerebral functioning is normally under the control of the upper hemispheric structures, the persistence of these same reflexes becomes pathological. However, the time required for these primitive reflexes to disappear varies substantially, and this must be taken into account when scoring. Evaluating primitive reflexes is no longer beneficial after 9 months of age, with the exception of the asymmetric tonic neck reflex—often the only primitive reflex that shows subtle persistence.

If the infant is examined during the second or third month, the Moro, finger grasp, or automatic walking reflexes may already be absent if the child's development has been particularly advanced and rapid. Therefore, the absence of these three reflexes should not be considered abnormal except in a clinical case of CNS depression.

Sucking

TECHNIQUE

Non-nutritive sucking is easily analyzed by inserting the examiner's little finger curled downward on the middle part of the tongue. This contact alone stimulates the sucking reflex. Sucking is not a continuous phenomenon; it includes bursts of movements separated by rest periods. In the full-term infant, there are usually eight or more sucking movements in a burst; the rhythm is rapid and bursts last for five to six seconds. A strong negative pressure is felt (infant sucks the finger) when facial motility is normal, ensuring a good seal of the lips over the finger.

SCORING

- Circle 0 if characteristics of normal sucking are present (rhythmic movements with adequate negative pressure).

- Circle 1 if the number of repetitions and negative pressure are insufficient.

- Circle 2 if sucking is absent or completely inadequate (owing to lack of closure of the infant's mouth on the examiner's finger or weak tongue movements).

Moro Reflex

TECHNIQUE

With the child lying in a dorsal decubitus position, the examiner gently raises the child a few centimeters off the table by both hands, with the infant's upper limbs in extension. When the examiner quickly lets go of the child's hands, the child falls back onto the examination table and the Moro reflex appears. The first observation is abduction of the arms with extension of the forearms (arms open), followed by adduction of the arms and flexion of the forearms (arms embrace). During the first part of the reflex, the infant's hands open completely. Crying and an anxious expression are part of the response.

SCORING

- Circle 0 if the Moro reflex is present during the first three months.
- Circle 2 if this reflex is present after 6 months of age.
- The presence of this reflex is insignificant between 3 and 6 months of age and is indicated with an "X."

Grasping Reflex of the Fingers

TECHNIQUE

The examiner places his or her index fingers in the palms of the infant's hands. This palmar stimulation causes strong flexion of the fingers, known as the *grasping reflex*. This maneuver can evaluate both hands at the same time.

SCORING

- Circle 0 if the grasping reflex is present during the first three months.
- Circle 2 if this reflex is present after 6 months of age.
- The presence of this reflex is insignificant between 3 and 6 months of age and is indicated with an "X."

The examiner will be able to lift the infant once he or she has grasped the examiner's fingers. This is made possible as the response spreads to all of the flexor muscles in the upper limbs. Once lifted off the examination table, the infant can support all or part of his or her own weight. If the infant is very alert and participating well in the examination, his or her head will pass through the body axis and the flexed lower limbs will lift up. This maneuver is more spectacular than useful because it is caused by a primitive reflex (grasping) and a stretch reflex of the flexor muscles of the upper limbs, which contract in response to rapid stretching. However, since the harmonious nature of the motor reflex involves the whole body, and since this maneuver can be perfectly performed only when the infant is very alert and interacting well with the examiner, this manipulation (called *response to traction*) remains a good indicator of the optimal state of the neonate.

Automatic Walking Reflex

TECHNIQUE

In the first few months, the infant is held in a vertical position, the examiner placing one hand in the upper thoracic region, with the thumb and middle finger under each armpit (the index finger is kept free to prevent the head from moving too much, if necessary). After the first few months, the infant is held in a vertical position by placing one hand under each armpit. The examiner observes the straightening of the legs and trunk. The infant should support most of his or her own body weight for a few seconds. The infant is then gently tilted forward and should take a few steps.

NOTE

Automatic walking implies a rhythmic contraction of the antigravity muscles elicited by cutaneous contact on the sole of the foot. Newborns can climb up stairs but cannot climb down stairs.

- Circle 0 if the automatic walking reflex is present during the first three months.

- Circle 2 if this reflex is present after 6 months of age.

- The presence of this reflex is insignificant between 3 and 6 months of age and is indicated with an "X."

Asymmetric Tonic Neck Reflex (ATNR) (or Fencing Posture)

TECHNIQUE

During the first few months, spontaneous asymmetric tonic neck reflex (ATNR) can be observed when the infant is lying in a dorsal decubitus position. If the infant's head is rotated to either side, a particular posture of the limbs is observed. In its obvious form (Fig. 15), the infant extends the upper limb on the side toward which his or her face is turned (facial side) and flexes the upper limb of the opposite side (occipital side). A similar but less prominent response may also be elicited in the lower limbs. This posture is called *evident ATNR* (see the examination chart). Like other primitive reflexes, this fencing posture (facial arm extended and occipital arm flexed) is normal in preterm and full-term newborns during the first few months of life. After the age of 6 months, evident ATNR is a sign of insufficient upper control over subcortical cerebral function. It remains present in severe CP and seriously restricts voluntary motor activity.

After 4 years of age, subtle persistence of this posture is evaluated. (Before 4 years, this reflex is too difficult to elicit because the child does not understand the instructions.) The child is placed on hands and knees with arms extended. To avoid the elbows being locked in extension, the child's hands are turned inward, with fingers facing each other. The examiner passively rotates the child's head. Normally, this passive rotation does not change the support of the arms and they remain extended. If flexing of the occipital arm is observed (Fig. 16),

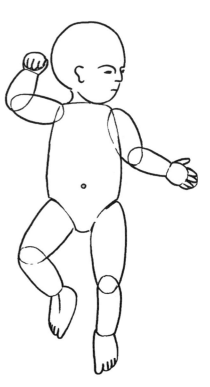

FIG. 15. SPONTANEOUS/EVIDENT
ASYMMETRIC TONIC NECK REFLEX
(ATNR)
During the first few months, this reflex is
observed with the child in the decubitus
dorsal position. The fencing posture (occipital arm flexed, facial arm extended)
indicates that passive tone of the limbs is
not yet independent of the position of
the head.

ATNR is present, but it will barely, if at all, interfere with voluntary motor activity. In the chart, a positive result is noted as *elicited ATNR*.

SCORING

- Circle 0 if ATNR is absent at 6 months of age.

- Circle 2 if ATNR is markedly present after 6 months.

> NOTE
> Strong deep tendon reflexes, the Babinski sign, and primitive reflexes are not abnormal in the newborn or during the first few months. The very young infant can be described at this age as "physiologically spastic."

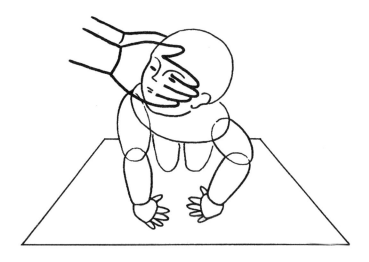

FIG. 16. ELICITED ASYMMETRIC TONIC NECK REFLEX (ATNR)
With the infant on all fours (arms extended, head in the axis), the examiner
passively rotates the head. If this maneuver causes the occipital arm to flex, the
ATNR reflex is still present.

- Circle 1 if, after the age of 4 years, flexing of the occipital arm is observed when the infant is on all fours (elicited ATNR).

Before 6 months of age, the presence or absence of this reflex is insignificant and is indicated with an "X."

Right/Left Asymmetry in Primitive Reflexes

Asymmetry in reflex responses can be observed when responses are
normally present at the infant's age (i.e., scored 0). In this case, the examiner should indicate the affected side (sluggish or absent response).
Asymmetry is particularly observed in the Moro reflex and the grasping reflex.

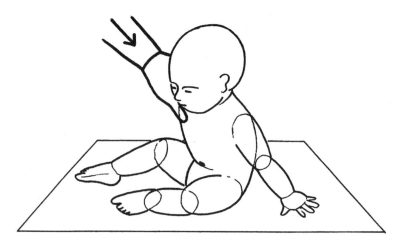

FIG. 17. LATERAL PROPPING REACTION (WHILE SEATED)
When the sitting child receives a brisk push at shoulder level, he or she avoids falling by extending the opposite arm.

Postural Reactions

Postural reactions appear during the first year in response to rapid movements felt by the infant. Once they appear, they persist throughout life. The absence of postural reactions is interpreted according to age.

Lateral Propping Reaction While Seated

TECHNIQUE

With the infant sitting independently, the examiner briskly pushes the child laterally at shoulder level. The child should extend his or her arm to the opposite side to avoid falling (Fig. 17). This postural reaction is elicited only after a solid sitting position is acquired. It is normally present between 6 and 8 months of age, as soon as the child can sit independently, and is therefore not tested during the first six months.

- Circle 0 if the lateral propping reaction is present from 6 months of age.

- Circle 1 if this reaction is incomplete between 9 and 24 months.

- Circle 2 if this reaction is absent after 9 months (even if the test cannot be performed because of the child's inability to sit independently) or if the response is incomplete after 24 months.

If the lateral propping reaction is incomplete or absent between 6 and 9 months of age, this cannot be interpreted and the examiner should circle "X."

Parachute Reaction

TECHNIQUE

While held in a ventral suspension position against the examiner's body, the child is quickly pushed with the head forward toward the examination table. The infant should rapidly extend the upper limbs with open hands, as if to protect himself or herself from falling (Fig. 18). This reaction appears in a precise form only between 8 and 9 months and is therefore not tested during the first six months.

SCORING

- Circle 0 if the parachute reaction is present from 6 months of age.

- Circle 1 if this reaction is incomplete between 9 and 24 months or absent between 9 and 12 months.

> NOTE
> The parachute reaction is very useful in daily life for catching one's balance, which is why it is dangerous for people to walk with their hands in their pockets.

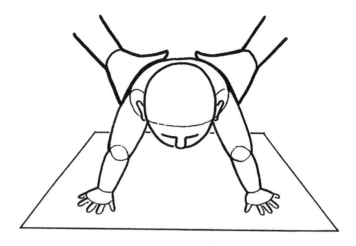

FIG. 18. PARACHUTE REACTION (FORWARD)

The child is quickly pushed forward toward the examination table; the child protects himself or herself by extending both arms and opening both hands.

- Circle 2 if this reaction is absent after 12 months or incomplete after 24 months.

If the parachute reaction is incomplete or absent between 6 and 9 months, this cannot be interpreted and the examiner should circle "X."

Qualitative Abnormalities in Gross Motor Function and Acquired Deformities

Certain abnormal signs preceding the acquisition of a motor function are interesting to note since they often provide clues about the most likely pathophysiological mechanism. However, these signs can also be misleading and cause the examiner to wrongly conclude that a motor function has been acquired. The most common examples are analyzed and scored, if necessary, according to age. Only after 2 years of age (examinations VII, VIII, IX, and X) does scoring become more precise.

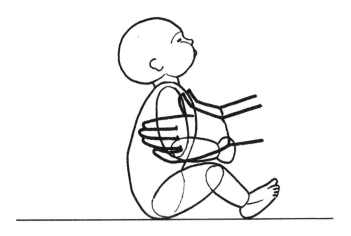

FIG. 19. HEAD HELD BEHIND THE AXIS BY HYPERTONIC OR
SHORTENED TRAPEZIUS MUSCLES

Head control seems to be present, but the head is not in the axis and the chin
points upward. At the nape of the neck, the trapezius muscles feel short and
stiff.

Head Control

Holding the Head behind the Axis. Head control behind the axis com-
monly occurs during the first six months. The head does not fall forward when the trunk is leaned forward, and the chin points upward
in a typical chin-forward position (Fig. 19). The examiner can feel that
the trapezius muscles are short and stiff. This false control of the head
can be the result of hypertonia of the extensors (a CNS problem) or
shortening of the trapezius muscles due to abnormal postures. Because
the interpretation is uncertain, head control behind the axis is not
scored before 2 years of age.

After 2 years and depending on the circumstances, the CNS nature of
this sign is easier to establish and is scored on the examination chart.

SCORING

- Circle 0 if head control behind the axis is absent.

- Circle 2 if this abnormality is present.

Before 2 years of age, the presence of this abnormality is indicated with an "X."

Poorly Maintained Head Control Due to Fatigue. Poor head control when fatigued is an indicator of a partial disability affecting both the flexors and the extensors. The child can voluntarily lift his or her head on request, but can support it for only a relatively short time owing to fatigue or lack of attention. This abnormality is not scored before 2 years of age. If still present after 2 years, the significance of this abnormality is very serious.

SCORING

- Circle 0 if poor head control when fatigued is absent.

- Circle 2 if this abnormality is present.

Before 2 years of age, the presence of this abnormality is indicated with an "X."

Sitting Position

Failure to Sit Due to Falling Forward. At this most insignificant stage in the acquisition of independent sitting, falling forward is a result of a certain degree of axial hypotonia. It is not scored until 9 months of age (because it is a simple exaggeration of a physiological phenomenon).

SCORING

- Circle 0 if failure to sit due to falling forward is absent.

- Circle 1 if this abnormality is present between 9 and 12 months of age.

- Circle 2 if this abnormality is present after 12 months.

Between 6 and 9 months of age, the presence of this abnormality is indicated with an "X."

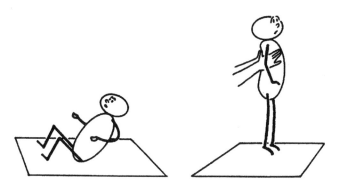

FIG. 20. FALLING BACKWARD WHEN SITTING AND EXCESSIVE
EXTENSION WHILE STANDING

These abnormalities are often linked together and are an indication of a lack
of upper control. (The mother indicates that her child cannot maintain a sitting position and always wants to stand.) (Reprinted with permission from
C. Amiel-Tison and A. Grenier. *Neurological Assessment during the First Year of Life*.
New York: Oxford University Press; 1986.)

Failure to Sit Due to Falling Backward. Falling backward is caused
partly by an inability to adopt the tripod position because hypertonia
of the flexor and adductor muscles in the legs keeps the knees too high
and close to one another, and partly by unbalanced axial tone in favor
of the extensor muscles. Falling backward is therefore unavoidable
(Fig. 20). The presence of this abnormality is scored from 6 months of
age (because it is not an exaggeration of a physiological phenomenon).

SCORING

- Circle 0 if failure to sit due to falling backward is absent.

- Circle 1 if this abnormality is present between 6 and 12 months of
  age.

- Circle 2 if this abnormality is present after 12 months.

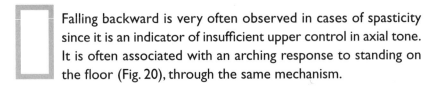

Falling backward is very often observed in cases of spasticity since it is an indicator of insufficient upper control in axial tone. It is often associated with an arching response to standing on the floor (Fig. 20), through the same mechanism.

Poorly Maintained Sitting Position Due to Fatigue. Poor maintenance of the sitting position when fatigued has the same significance as that indicated for head control when fatigued. It is scored after 2 years of age.

SCORING

- Circle 0 if poor sitting due to fatigue is absent.

- Circle 2 if this abnormality is present after 2 years of age.

Before 2 years of age, the presence of this abnormality is indicated with an "X."

Acquired Deformities. Scoliosis is a common complication of CP in cases of unilateral or predominantly unilateral lesions, according to the distribution of paralysis, spasticity, and orthopedic problems in the pelvic region and lower limbs. This deformity is scored after 2 years of age.

SCORING

- Circle 0 if scoliosis is absent.

- Circle 1 if this deformity is present after 2 years of age.

Kyphosis is a common deformity caused by spasticity and the shortening of the hamstring muscles. When in a sitting position, the ischium slides forward to draw the hamstring insertions closer together. Kyphosis worsens when the child is seated on the floor. This deformity is scored after 2 years of age.

- Circle 0 if kyphosis is absent.

- Circle 1 if this deformity is present after 2 years of age.

Standing Position

Excessive Extension While Standing. Excessive extension while standing is an excessive reaction of the antigravity muscles that creates an opisthotonos (or arched) posture. This is abnormal at any age (Fig. 20).

SCORING

- Circle 0 if arched posture while standing is absent.

- Circle 2 if this deformity is present.

Lower Limb Deformities. Scissoring of the lower limbs, crossing of the legs in extension, is most often associated with an equine deformity of the foot, making standing difficult. The presence of scissoring is abnormal at any age.

SCORING

- Circle 0 if scissoring of the lower limbs is absent.

- Circle 2 if this deformity is present.

> Scissoring is a strong indicator of spastic diplegia. One symptom of spastic diplegia is spasticity in the adductor muscles of the thigh. However, early shortening of these muscles due to abnormal postures in the neonatal period most often precedes spasticity. In the absence of immediate attention in the intensive care unit, scissoring is partly a sign of a posture-induced deformity and partly a symptom of a CNS disorder due to a lack of upper control.

Some additional lower limb deformities include the following:

Permanent flexion of the hip: a limitation of full extension.

Permanent flexion of the knee: a limitation of full extension.

Equine deformity of the foot: a permanent and irreducible extension of the foot.

Dislocation of the hip: a serious complication of spasticity that should be prevented by adapted positioning from birth.

The presence of each of these deformities is indicated with an "X."

Only the most common deformities have been mentioned here. Other abnormal standing postures should be clearly described according to dystonic muscle groups and acquired muscular shortenings.

Gait

Only a clinical analysis of walking (not a laboratory assessment) is included in the examination chart. Gait analysis requires keen observation for defining specific types of limping. The most common of these abnormalities observed in infants with CP are the following:

Spastic gait: linked to spasticity in the antigravity muscles with toe-walking and lifting of the body each time the foot touches the floor (skipping).

Ataxic gait: linked to a balance problem with broad-based stance and frequent falls.

NOTE
With immediate and constant adapted positioning of the child from birth, "classical" spastic diplegia becomes "modern" diplegia or diplegia without scissoring.

Hemiplegic gait: linked to a muscular disability that makes the child circumduct a leg (like a scythe).

Walking with assistance (tripod, walker, etc.): this should also be noted.

The presence of each of these abnormalities is indicated with an "X."

Chapter 4

Clinical Profiles According to Age

- Step-by-Step Profiles up to 2 Years
- Short-Term Profile at 2 Years (Corrected Age)
- Annual Profiles up to 6 Years

Step-by-Step Profiles up to 2 Years

General Comments

The detailed descriptions and scoring instructions for each observation or maneuver of the pediatric neurological examination (as given
in Chapter 3) increase objectivity and promote the use of a common
language. This analytical approach is the basis of all neurological follow-ups. However, using this information is not as simple as it may
seem, because the data from three age periods (before, at, and after the
age of 2 years) must be treated differently.

Before 2 Years of Age. Examiners must be extremely careful when interpreting the scoring results of a single examination in children under
2 years of age. As we have seen, individuals vary greatly in muscle tone
and motor development. What should examiners do about abnormalities observed during the first two years of life? Some sound advice
is to conduct step-by-step profiles based on groupings, or clusters, of
abnormalities.

To analyze and define these clusters, examiners must use the scores of
0, 1, and 2 recorded in each section of the examination chart for the
first six examinations (I to VI) to gather together the most important
signs and symptoms.

1. *For each section:* Examiners should assign the highest score to the
   entire section—that is, individual scores for each item are not
   summed.

2. *Overall interpretation of the examination at each age period:* Severe
   deficit is defined by the predominance of a score of 2 based on the
   total number of sections indicated in the tables in this chapter (Tables 1 to 4). Moderate deficit is defined by the predominance of a
   score of 1 based on the total number of sections indicated in each
   table. Note that a few scores of 2 are acceptable for the moderate
   deficit category.

These profiles serve as provisional conclusions for medical records, allowing precise indications for possible interventions. The profiles

should not be used in any other way for children under 2 years of age. This is why the profiles described in the tables are not incorporated in the examination chart. Any system based on calculation of an overall score would result in distorted interpretations of neurological or maturative events. The purpose of analyzing these successive abnormal profiles is to identify a trend rather than a cut-off point.

Only the most frequent and typical clinical profiles are described here. The following criteria are taken into account for each age period:

1. The nature of the observed neuromotor abnormalities, their grouping, and their functional consequences.

2. The fixed nature or progressive trend of the observed signs (described as *static* or *dynamic*).

3. The emergence of specific neuromotor signs with cerebral maturation.

4. Concomitant changes in brain growth, as evidenced by measurement of head circumference (HC) growth and examination of the fontanels and cranial sutures.

5. The detection of related sensory or cognitive deviations or epilepsy.

During the first nine months, observed signs are still nonspecific. In other words, with the exception of extensive and severe brain damage, this is a "wait and see" period. Great care must be exercised in discussions with parents during this time.

At approximately 9 months of age, neuromotor abnormalities become specific and related sensory or cognitive deviations become progressively more evident.

So as to remain simple in our descriptions of some of the most typical profiles, we assume that prevention of secondary muscular shortening by adapted positioning has been successfully applied from the first day of life and pursued thereafter. In other words, the current results of the neuromotor examination are not, or at least are only slightly, contaminated by secondary orthopedic consequences of the CNS insult (particularly for the trapezius in the upper limbs and adductor muscles in the lower limbs).

At 2 Years (Corrected Age). At 2 years of age the situation becomes clearer. Children with neurological signs who have not acquired the ability to walk independently are diagnosed as having cerebral palsy (CP). A symptomatic and topographical diagnosis, as well as an etiological diagnosis (if possible), allows the analysis of short-term results for a cohort of children.

After 2 Years of Age. Annual profiles allow further clarification about the severity of neuromotor dysfunction in children with CP and an evaluation of related abnormalities of cerebral functions other than neuromotor function.

Classification for children 2 years of age and the annual profiles are found on page 18 of the examination chart. Follow-ups should be continued until the age of learning disabilities for children who show persisting neurological abnormalities even though they have not been diagnosed as having CP (because they walked before the age of 2 years). These children are also included on page 18 of the chart.

First Trimester—Neonatal Period and First Three Months of Life

At the end of the first three months of life, a provisional profile permits the clinician to determine two clinical characteristics: *severe deficit* and *moderate deficit*. The characteristics of severe and moderate deficits are summarized in Table 1. If these children could be examined repeatedly throughout the first few weeks and months of life, another clinical characteristic could be determined: *static* or *dynamic profile*.

Static Profile. A static neurological profile of CP is defined by little observable change during the first weeks after birth. Signs already present at birth change very little during the following weeks, suggesting the damage occurred before birth (Fig. 21). Certain signs present from the first few days of life—including cortical thumb, high-arched palate, and overlapping cranial sutures (Fig. 22)—serve as strong indicators that the insult is of prenatal origin. It is very important that these signs

TABLE I
Definition of Severe and Moderate Deficits at the End of Three Months

Sections	Severe Deficit	Moderate Deficit
Head growth (HC, growth profile, fontanels and sutures)	2	1
Social interaction (alertness and attention, visual tracking, excitability)	2	1
Passive muscle tone (limbs and trunk)	2	1
Motor activity (quality and quantity)	2	1
Primitive reflexes (absent or insufficient, especially sucking)	2	1

Note: Severe deficit: a score of 2 in at least four of five sections. Moderate deficit: mostly scores of 1; some scores of 2 are acceptable in this category.

be noted immediately because they soon lose their significance in allowing a precise determination of the chronology of events.

Dynamic Profile. A dynamic neurological profile of CP is defined by rapid improvement, especially in alertness, sucking, swallowing, and

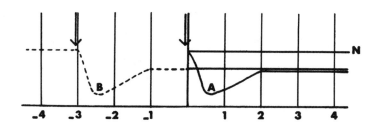

FIG. 21. CHANGING PROFILES DURING THE FIRST WEEKS OF LIFE
Negative numbers indicate weeks before birth; positive numbers indicate weeks after birth. N: normal profile, no CNS depression. A: dynamic profile secondary to a recent lesion, occurring around birth. CNS depression worsens, then stabilizes. B: static profile secondary to a prenatal lesion. CNS depression is already stabilized at birth, the acute stage having preceded birth. (Reprinted with permission from C. Amiel-Tison. Correlations between hypoxic-ischemic events during fetal life and outcome. In: P. Arbeille, D. Maulik, R. Laurini, eds. *Fetal Hypoxia.* London: Parthenon Press; 1999.)

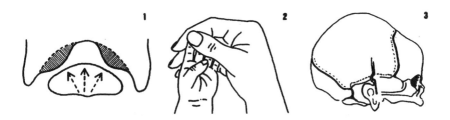

FIG. 22. NEONATAL SIGNS INDICATING A PRENATAL INSULT
Shown here are 1: high-arched palate; 2: cortical thumb; 3: overlapping sutures. These three signs are often associated. When present at birth, they indicate a lesion that is several or more weeks old. (Reprinted with permission from C. Amiel-Tison. Correlations between hypoxic-ischemic events during fetal life and outcome. In: P. Arbeille, D. Maulik, R. Laurini, eds. *Fetal Hypoxia.* London: Parthenon Press; 1999.)

spontaneous movements. In the weeks following a serious event such as an epileptic seizure, a return of the ability to suck efficiently well to take in adequate amounts of nutrition has always been considered an indicator of a favorable outcome: a return of this ability at the end of the first week is a good sign; a return at the end of the third week or later is a poor sign; a return during the in-between period is difficult to interpret. The dynamic profile indicates that the lesion occurred very close to birth. Following a moderate deficit, a rapid improvement, which after a few weeks results in optimum alertness and acquisition of head control (typically acquired at 2 months of age), indicates a favorable outcome.

Head Circumference Growth. Growth in HC is an important factor in defining static and dynamic profiles.

NOTE
There is little evidence of neurological development during the first three months until head control is acquired. Perfect control of the head in the axis is a major event often ignored in medical records, and likewise not often remembered by parents.

A typical situation in CP with a static neurological profile is an HC measurement that is already lower on the growth curves than other growth parameters. This situation remains the same during the following few weeks and months, without catching up.

A typical situation in CP with a dynamic neurological profile is an initially normal HC measurement, possibly followed by a secondary decline in the rate of growth.

Unclassified Minor Abnormalities. Some abnormalities are not included in Table 1 because of their heterogeneity; they include hyperexcitability and various abnormalities in muscle tone. The most common minor abnormalities are associated with excessive motor activity, insufficient sleep, inconsolable excessive crying, tremors, clonic movements, and a tendency toward muscular hypertonia. The absence of alertness-related problems and the lack of primitive reflex depression are important factors in arguing against CNS depression, establishing the difference between these minor abnormalities and the moderate deficits described in Table 1. The most frequent trend is toward normalization, in a few weeks or a few months.

Second Trimester—From 4 to 6 Months of Age

At the end of six months, the provisional profile consists of two clinical aspects: severe and moderate deficits (described in Table 2). In most cases, abnormalities remain nonspecific and include signs similar to those seen in the first three months, but they tend to cluster with other abnormalities indicating a deficit in upper motor control. The cephalocaudal (descending) wave of relaxation does not progress to the limbs. Insufficient progress of active muscle tone in the neck flexors results in the absence of head control before 4 months of age. Lastly, cranial signs often manifest as a decline in the rate of head growth or as ridges at cranial sutures. In the most severe cases only, an unfavorable outcome may appear unavoidable at the end of six months, based on the following indicators:

TABLE 2
Definition of Severe and Moderate Deficits between Four and Six Months

Sections	Severe Deficit	Moderate Deficit
Head growth (HC, growth profile, fontanels and sutures)	2	1
Social interaction (alertness and attention, visual tracking, excitability)	2	1
Passive muscle tone (limbs and trunk)	2	1
Motor activity (quality and quantity)	2	1
Primitive reflexes (sucking difficulties only)	2	1

Note: Severe deficit: a score of 2 in at least four of five sections. Moderate deficit: mostly scores of 1; some scores of 2 are acceptable in this category.

1. A marked decline in the rate of head growth

2. Specific neuromotor abnormalities, already suggesting CP

3. Infantile spasms (West syndrome)

Third Trimester—From 7 to 9 Months of Age

At this stage of development, neuromotor abnormalities become more specific and related disabilities (especially cognitive and sensory impairments) become more evident. However, related disabilities are not

---

NOTE
The second three-month period of life represents a time of hesitation and hope for pediatricians, because maturation can lead to the acquisition of skills despite neurological abnormalities. Examiners who primarily see children with severe brain injury in their practice can forget how amazing normal development looks.

TABLE 3

Definition of Severe and Moderate Deficits between Seven and Nine Months

Sections	Severe Deficit	Moderate Deficit
Head growth (HC, growth profile, fontanels and sutures)	2	I
Social interaction (alertness and attention, visual tracking, excitability)	2	I
Passive muscle tone (limbs and trunk)	2	I
Motor activity (quality and quantity)	2	I
Head control (scored according to age of acquisition)	2	I
Evident ATNR	2	0

Note: Severe deficit: a score of 2 in at least four of six sections. Moderate deficit: a score of I in at least four of six sections; some scores of 2 are acceptable in this category.

yet included in the provisional profile (as outlined in Table 3) because they are usually uncertain.

Severe Deficit. Neuromotor abnormalities can already be characterized according to the predominance of major hypotonia or spasticity or rigidity, which most often affects all four limbs and the trunk. In many cases, in which any hope of normalization has disappeared, the diagnosis of CP may already be possible.

Moderate Deficit. At this age, it is almost impossible to differentiate between the onset of spastic diplegia and a specific set of "spastic-like" symptoms. If the descending wave of relaxation does not progress normally to the limbs and if antigravity reactions are still marked, this indicates a problem in the establishment of upper motor control. However, examiners must be very careful before deciding on the diagnosis of spastic diplegia (Little's disease) because the spastic-like symptoms may disappear quite abruptly at 9 months of age as a result of maturation. The child will be able to walk before 2 years of age, but this does not mean that all traces of minor cerebral damage have disappeared.

Fourth Trimester—From 10 to 12 Months of Age and during the Second Year

Severe or Moderate Neurological Deficits. If severe or moderate abnormalities are present at the end of the first year, they will remain permanently. Several factors influence the severity of these deficits during the second year:

1. Functional consequences, when the child is well past the normal age for acquiring head control and independent sitting skills.

2. Orthopedic consequences of spasticity and rigidity—that is, muscular shortening and bone/joint deformities—despite attempts to prevent these by the orthopedist and physical therapist.

3. The association of involuntary movements and dystonia, which affect voluntary movements.

4. The association of nonmotor deficits (i.e., communication, development of prelanguage, vision, hearing).

5. Seizures.

These factors, outlined in Table 4, allow examiners to differentiate between severe, moderate, and mild deficits during the second year of life.

Minor Neurological Anomalies. Passive overextension of the trunk is generally noticed in the first months of life and remains unchanged. A *squamous ridge* may also appear early in life and may still be present at 2 years of age (though it may disappear over the next few years as the skull remolds itself). In addition, mild distal spasticity may appear during the second year only, most often revealed as a *phasic stretch of the triceps surae during rapid dorsiflexion of the foot*; the later it appears, the milder it is considered to be. Since this type of spasticity often goes unrecognized, it can eventually lead to a slight muscle and tendon shortening. (A slow 90° angle will have little or no effect on walking but will make running difficult.) For these children, the ability to walk independently will be acquired slightly late—either within acceptable normal limits (before 18 months) or between 18 months and 2 years.

TABLE 4
Definition of Severe, Moderate, and Minor Deficits between 10 and 24 Months

Sections	Severe Deficit	Moderate Deficit	Minor Abnormality
Head growth (insufficient HC growth; all sutures abnormal or an isolated abnormality with squamous sutures)	2	1 or 2	0 or 1
Social interaction (alertness and attention, visual tracking, excitability)	2	1	0
Passive muscle tone (limbs and trunk)			
Trunk imbalance	2	1	1
Stretch reflex in limbs	2	1 or 2	1
Hypotonia or rigidity	2	0	0
Involuntary movements	2	0	0
Parachute reaction (scored according to age of acquisition)	2	1	0
Gross motor skills (scored according to age of acquisition)			
Head control	2	1	0
Sitting position	2	1	0
Independent walking	1	1	0 or 1

Note: Severe deficit: a score of 2 in at least six of seven sections (including the inability to walk). Moderate deficit: a score of 1 in at least five of seven sections; some scores of 2 are acceptable in this category. Minor abnormality: a score of 1 in at least three of seven sections.

> NOTE
> In favorable cases, only these three neurological and cranial signs remain at the end of the first year. On rare occasions, the phasic stretch appears during the second year. Examiners must therefore continue a systematic search for this sign.

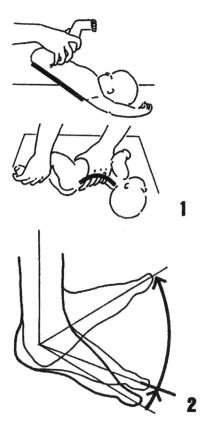

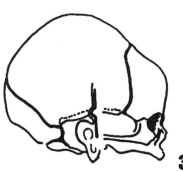

FIG. 23. INDICATORS OF A MINOR PERINATAL LESION
Shown here are *1*: imbalance in passive muscle tone of the trunk with excessive extension; *2*: phasic stretch during rapid dorsiflexion of the foot; *3*: squamous ridge (may disappear after the age of 2 years). These three signs (or at least the first two) are only significant when clustered together. (Reprinted with permission from C. Amiel-Tison. Correlations between hypoxic-ischemic events during fetal life and outcome. In: P. Arbeille, D. Maulik, R. Laurini, eds. *Fetal Hypoxia*. London: Parthenon Press; 1999.)

These three abnormalities, which appear early in life or during the second year, form a triad of symptoms (Fig. 23) that serve as indicators for monitoring the child's future development, and thus are part of the profile for the second year of life (Table 4). These mild signs are particularly relevant when they are found together, as a cluster.

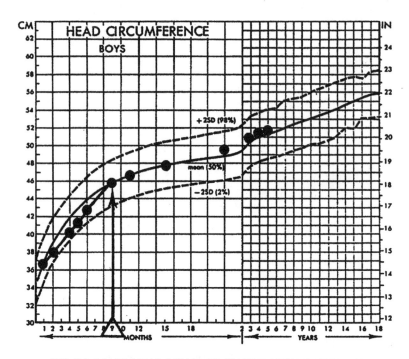

FIG. 24. ABNORMAL HEAD GROWTH WITH CATCH UP

This diagram shows a moderate decline in growth, followed by a catch up at 9 months of age. Measurements are recorded on the Nelhaus Growth Chart (for boys). (Reprinted with permission from G. Nelhaus. *Pediatrics* 1968;41:106-112.)

Head Growth Abnormalities. After 2 years of age, abnormalities in skull development permit the observation of several gradual profiles:

1. Relative microcephaly (compared with other growth parameters) or absolute microcephaly (−2 SD) observed at birth and persisting after birth, attributable to prenatal lesions.

2. Relative or absolute microcephaly observed later (during the first six months), attributable to perinatal lesions and resulting in an abnormal head growth profile without catch up.

3. Moderate decline in the rate of head growth, followed by a catch up. A period of "inertia" from 2 to 3 months of age is followed by stabilization for a few months at about −1 SD, then a catch up at the

end of the first year (Fig. 24). This profile is often associated with the minor neurological abnormalities described above.

Other Specific Clinical Syndromes

Unilateral Impairment. Unilateral impairment is easily observed clinically at an early age. With the normal side of the body used as the control for evaluation of passive tone in the limbs, the large variability within normal limits is therefore neutralized. The challenge at this period is to determine which side of the body is abnormal; this is not always obvious in the first few months. The signs of spastic hemiplegia develop in the same way as signs of spastic diplegia: an initial phase of CNS depression leads to hypotonia, which in a few months is followed by the onset of spasticity. If the lesion (most often a prenatal infarction of the middle cerebral artery) is very recent, occurring shortly before birth, the abnormal side is the hypotonic side at first. A few months later, the abnormal side becomes the hypertonic side, with spasticity and increased deep tendon reflexes. However, if the prenatal lesion occurred several months before birth, the abnormal side is already hypertonic at birth.

- *A suggestion:* For the best guarantee of objectivity, it is advisable not to look at the brain imaging before conducting the examination.

- *An observation:* Although still often referred to in the literature on congenital hemiplegia, an interval between lesion and signs is rare. Abnormalities will change, but they are present from the first weeks of life.

- *A remark:* Spastic hemiplegia is classified as a clinical variety of CP even though independent walking is most often observed before 2 years of age (between 18 and 20 months, on average). This is a reasonable departure from the norm. The dysfunction predominates in the upper limb, while moderate spasticity in the lower limb often permits relatively normal gait.

Benign Congenital Hypotonia. Benign congenital hypotonia often causes examiners some hesitation in making a diagnosis during the first few months. Passive tone is very relaxed throughout the body, while active tone is sufficient. Independent sitting is acquired within normal time limits, yet walking is often delayed (to shortly before or shortly after 18 months). The diagnosis of benign congenital hypotonia is based on two factors: observation of the absolutely isolated characteristics of the muscle tone problem and an interview with the parents to determine whether any family members have the same hypotonia, which may still be present at an advanced age, but with no other signs.

Short-Term Profile at 2 Years (Corrected Age)

Diagnosis of Cerebral Palsy

The diagnosis of CP is possible at 2 years of age when neuromotor abnormalities are serious enough to make independent walking impossible. The clinical subtype of CP can be confirmed at this time, because any neurological sign present at 2 years will persist throughout life. Only functional consequences will change, and other cerebral functional deficits will possibly interfere with motor function. For topography and symptomatology, examiners should clearly indicate the clinical subtype on the profile summary sheet (page 18 of the examination chart).

Topographical Classifications

Topographical variations of spasticity are described in Table 5.

Symptomatic Clusters

Spastic Cerebral Palsy. Pyramidal signs predominate in spastic CP. These signs include spasticity (abnormal response to rapid stretching), exaggerated deep tendon reflexes, and the Babinski sign, but few if any involuntary movements.

TABLE 5
Topographical Classifications of Spastic Cerebral Palsy

Hemiplegia	Affects upper and lower limbs on the same side, especially upper limb
Diplegia	Affects all four limbs, but mainly lower limbs
Quadriplegia	Affects all four limbs equally
Double hemiplegia	Affects all four limbs, but mainly upper limbs
Monoplegia	Most often affects upper limbs (often part of a hemiplegia with almost normal function of lower limbs)
Triplegia	A probable variant of quadriplegia

Dyskinetic (or Hyperkinetic) Cerebral Palsy. Dyskinetic CP is defined by diffuse rigidity and involuntary movements, which interfere with the child's (very limited) voluntary movement. Subtypes of dyskinetic CP depend on the nature of the associated movements rather than their topography, because all four limbs and the face are affected. Motor function is severely affected.

Ataxic Cerebral Palsy. Ataxic CP is characterized by a broad-based stance, unsteadiness of the trunk, frequent falls, dysmetria, and abnormal eye movements. Muscle tone is hypotonic throughout the body. Pure ataxic CP is rare and indicates the need for clinical investigation into a cerebellar disorder, most often genetic in origin.

Mixed-Type Cerebral Palsy. Mixed CP occurs frequently, as opposed to extrapyramidal CP, which does not. It is common to find subtle signs of spasticity and rigidity in a "dyskinetic" child. It is also common for a "spastic" child to experience involuntary movements. There are, of course, countless variations of mixed CP, and this classification is left to the examiner.

THESE CATEGORIES OF CP ARE USEFUL because they indicate different pathophysiologies (either more pyramidal or more extrapyramidal in nature) as well as various etiologies and a distinct prognosis.

Classification of Cerebral Palsy according to Age Variations in the Ability or Inability to Walk Independently

Cerebral palsy can be classified into three levels depending on the ability to walk independently:

1. Ability to walk between 2 and 3 years of age: moderate deficit.

2. Ability to walk between 3 and 5 years: severe deficit.

3. Ability to walk independently still not acquired at 5 years: profound deficit.

Classification of Cerebral Palsy according to the Severity of Related Disabilities

The related disabilities can be cognitive, visual, or auditory, but can also include epilepsy or hydrocephalus. These disabilities are defined as moderate or severe based on all clinical data and complementary investigations.

Annual Profiles up to 6 Years

Cerebral Palsy

The diagnosis of CP established at the age of 2 years will not change. However, its effects on motor function do change, as do the related disabilities, which will have a variable impact on an individual's life as

---

NOTE

Examiners should never predict the time when a child will walk independently; even the most experienced examiners can be wrong. They should try to encourage parents not to put all their hope in the child's ability to walk.

---

a child and as an adult. These long-term aspects give the impression that this disorder evolves, even though, by definition, the cerebral lesion is nonprogressive.

Though not completely satisfactory, the label *cerebral palsy* does allow some distinctions between "central" and "peripheral" motor deficits (either neurological or muscular), on the one hand, and between predominantly motor and predominantly other central deficits (e.g., isolated mental deficiency, epilepsy, isolated sensory deficit, or even serious behavioral problems), on the other. These latter conditions are rarely due to hypoxic-ischemic lesions (as is CP) but are most often genetic. Consequently, such diagnoses are rarely made during long-term follow-ups of children considered at risk because of unfavorable circumstances at birth.

Moderate Neuromotor Abnormalities Compatible with Walking before 24 Months (Hemiplegia Excluded)

As previously discussed, the symptomatic triad of the following neurological and cranial signs can serve as a clue for interpreting learning problems:

1. A phasic stretch of both triceps surae, with increased deep tendon reflexes.

2. An imbalance of passive tone of the trunk, with more extension than flexion.

3. A palpable ridge at both squamous sutures.

NOTE
This symptomatic triad allows the detection of a group of children at risk for learning difficulties. These later dysfunctions are not guaranteed to occur, but they frequently do, and so interventions should be available to help these children.

These neuromotor abnormalities are permanent markers of perinatal lesions. The squamous ridge is the only abnormality that may disappear over time. Because these three signs are so subtle, they can be detected only through systematic neurological examinations. The purpose of this analysis is to permit further specialized follow-ups and future education-based intervention, since the risk of learning disabilities seems to be higher in this group than in the general population.

It is also interesting to note that these minor neurological signs are often present in children whose disabilities are mainly psychiatric. This is particularly true for many autistic children: neuromotor abnormalities are evident; the ability to walk is delayed (acquired, on average, near the age of 2 years); and, after 2 years of age, the abnormal behavior becomes the major sign. As these observations demonstrate, such psychiatric problems clearly point to a cerebral lesion.

Conclusion

The purpose of the evaluation tool presented in this book is to educate pediatricians and other health care professionals (such as occupational therapists and physical therapists) in the practice of neurological follow-ups. This practice enables health care practitioners to collect the results of repeated analytical examinations of children between birth and 6 years by using a single evaluation tool.

Once these results are collected, caregivers must begin to synthesize clinical profiles. Even if the identification of a typical abnormal profile is not possible, as is sometimes the case, the clustering of signs usually enables the examiner to follow a trend, which allows a diagnosis to be made at 2 years (corrected age).

Because this manual is limited to the explanation of a clinical tool, no complementary examinations have been included. However, the results of such assessments also form an integral part of the ultimate profile, and examiners can use additional protocol sheets if they wish.

The use of transfontanel ultrasound imaging plays a major role in pediatric neurological examinations. In preterm infants, assessing the extent of a lesion at 1 month of age is directly linked to prognosis for the long-term future, especially in cases of severe damage. However, the absence of damage visible by ultrasound imaging does not indicate that no damage exists. Obtaining normal ultrasound imaging results does not preclude systematic neurological follow-ups.

This manual is not intended to determine which results or observations should or should not be shared with the parents. Often the parents have seen the ultrasound imaging in the Neonatal Intensive Care Unit and have been informed about the probability of severe sequelae. Clinical follow-ups may indeed provide parents with some hope if the maturative changes are discussed in a positive manner. By temporarily withholding medical-based predictions, the pediatrician gives the child time to become part of the family. When it comes time to reveal the disappointing news (by the end of the first year), magnetic resonance imaging may help to give a more realistic estimation of the outcome.

The goal of these systematic examinations is to organize future intervention for the child: initial and subsequent orthopedic treatment in the case of CP, appropriate stimulation, neurodevelopmental rehabilitation, speech therapy, psychotherapy, special education, and so forth. All these interventions should precede specific diagnoses and allow for proper follow-up of child and family. Pediatricians rarely receive criticism from parents for a delayed announcement about neurological sequelae, as long as all the possible interventions have been provided.

Examination Chart

NEUROLOGICAL DEVELOPMENT FROM BIRTH TO 6 YEARS
CLAUDINE AMIEL-TISON AND JULIE GOSSELIN

PERSONAL INFORMATION

Name:	File No.:
Date of Birth:	Length of Gestation:

Examination		Date of Examination	Age	Corrected Age	Comments
1st–9th Month					
I	1st–3rd Month				
II	4th–6th Month				
III	7th–9th Month				
10th–24th Month					
IV	10th–12th Month				
V	13th–18th Month				
VI	19th–24th Month				
3rd–6th Year					
VII	3rd Year				
VIII	4th Year				
IX	5th Year				
X	6th Year				

Life Environment	Mother	Father
Date of Birth		
Education		
Profession		

Changes in the child's life during follow-up:

1

Growth			Head Circumference		Height		Weight		HC/Growth Discordance	
1st–9th Month										
I	HC:	cm	± 2 SD	0	± 2 SD	0	± 2 SD	0	HC is concordant	0
	Height:	cm	> 2 SD	2	> 2 SD	2	> 2 SD	2	Growth - related	
	Weight:	kg	< 2 SD	2	< 2 SD	2	< 2 SD	2	deficit of HC	X
II	HC:	cm	± 2 SD	0	± 2 SD	0	± 2 SD	0	HC is concordant	0
	Height:	cm	> 2 SD	2	> 2 SD	2	> 2 SD	2	Growth - related	
	Weight:	kg	< 2 SD	2	< 2 SD	2	< 2 SD	2	deficit of HC	X
III	HC:	cm	± 2 SD	0	± 2 SD	0	± 2 SD	0	HC is concordant	0
	Height:	cm	> 2 SD	2	> 2 SD	2	> 2 SD	2	Growth - related	
	Weight:	kg	< 2 SD	2	< 2 SD	2	< 2 SD	2	deficit of HC	X
10th–24th Month										
IV	HC:	cm	± 2 SD	0	± 2 SD	0	± 2 SD	0	HC is concordant	0
	Height:	cm	> 2 SD	2	> 2 SD	2	> 2 SD	2	Growth - related	
	Weight:	kg	< 2 SD	2	< 2 SD	2	< 2 SD	2	deficit of HC	X
V	HC:	cm	± 2 SD	0	± 2 SD	0	± 2 SD	0	HC is concordant	0
	Height:	cm	> 2 SD	2	> 2 SD	2	> 2 SD	2	Growth - related	
	Weight:	kg	< 2 SD	2	< 2 SD	2	< 2 SD	2	deficit of HC	X
VI	HC:	cm	± 2 SD	0	± 2 SD	0	± 2 SD	0	HC is concordant	0
	Height:	cm	> 2 SD	2	> 2 SD	2	> 2 SD	2	Growth - related	
	Weight:	kg	< 2 SD	2	< 2 SD	2	< 2 SD	2	deficit of HC	X
3rd–6th Year										
VII	HC:	cm	± 2 SD	0	± 2 SD	0	± 2 SD	0	HC is concordant	0
	Height:	cm	> 2 SD	2	> 2 SD	2	> 2 SD	2	Growth - related	
	Weight:	kg	< 2 SD	2	< 2 SD	2	< 2 SD	2	deficit of HC	X
VIII	HC:	cm	± 2 SD	0	± 2 SD	0	± 2 SD	0	HC is concordant	0
	Height:	cm	> 2 SD	2	> 2 SD	2	> 2 SD	2	Growth - related	
	Weight:	kg	< 2 SD	2	< 2 SD	2	< 2 SD	2	deficit of HC	X
IX	HC:	cm	± 2 SD	0	± 2 SD	0	± 2 SD	0	HC is concordant	0
	Height:	cm	> 2 SD	2	> 2 SD	2	> 2 SD	2	Growth - related	
	Weight:	kg	< 2 SD	2	< 2 SD	2	< 2 SD	2	deficit of HC	X
X	HC:	cm	± 2 SD	0	± 2 SD	0	± 2 SD	0	HC is concordant	0
	Height:	cm	> 2 SD	2	> 2 SD	2	> 2 SD	2	Growth - related	
	Weight:	kg	< 2 SD	2	< 2 SD	2	< 2 SD	2	deficit of HC	X

Head Growth Profile from 0 to 2 Years (Examinations I to VI)

Normal profile	0
Downward profile with catch up	X
Downward profile without catch up	X

2

Health Problems (Check appropriate boxes)

Health Problems (Check appropriate boxes)	I	II	III	IV	V	VI	VII	VIII	IX	X
Refraction disorder and/or retinopathy										
Transmission hearing loss										
Chronic pulmonary disease										
Chronic digestive problems										
Growth problems										
Malformation										
Other Specify: _____										

Craniofacial Examination

Craniofacial Examination	I	II	III	IV	V	VI	VII	VIII	IX	X
Ventriculo-peritoneal shunt										
Anterior fontanel Open	0	0	0	0						
Closed	2	2	2	1						
Sutures Edge-to-edge	0	0	0	0	0	0	0	0	0	0
Overlapping (ridge) Parietotemporal suture (squamous)	1	1	1	1	1	1	1	1	1	1
Frontal	1	1	1	1	1	1	1	1	1	1
Coronal	1	1	1	1	1	1	1	1	1	1
Sagittal	1	1	1	1	1	1	1	1	1	1
Occipital	1	1	1	1	1	1	1	1	1	1
Shape of skull Normal	0	0	0	0	0	0	0	0	0	0
Abnormal Describe:_____	1	1	1	1	1	1	1	1	1	1
Shape of palate Flat	0	0	0	0	0	0	0	0	0	0
High-arched	1	1	1	1	1	1	1	1	1	1

Neurosensory Examination	I	II	III	IV	V	VI	VII	VIII	IX	X
Hearing										
Normal	0	0	0	0	0	0	0	0	0	0
Moderate hearing loss	1	1	1	1	1	1	1	1	1	1
Profound hearing loss	2	2	2	2	2	2	2	2	2	2
Vision and ocular signs										
Fix and track										
Easy to obtain	0	0	0	0	0	0	0	0	0	0
Difficult to maintain	1	1	1	1	1	1	1	1	1	1
No response	2	2	2	2	2	2	2	2	2	2
Nystagmus										
Absent	0	0	0	0	0	0	0	0	0	0
Present	2	2	2	2	2	2	2	2	2	2
Eye movements										
Synchronous	0	0	0	0	0	0	0	0	0	0
Erratic	2	2	2	2	2	2	2	2	2	2
Strabismus										
Absent	0	0	0	0	0	0	0	0	0	0
Present	1	1	1	1	1	1	1	1	1	1
Sunset sign										
Absent	0	0	0	0	0	0	0	0	0	0
Present	2	2	2	2	2	2	2	2	2	2

Diagnostic tests

Hearing (audiogram, BAEP):

Vision (VEP, ERG):

Observations and Interview	I	II	III	IV	V	VI	VII	VIII	IX	X
Seizures										
Absent	0	0	0	0	0	0	0	0	0	0
Febrile seizures	X	X	X	X	X	X	X	X	X	X
Focal and/or easily controlled seizures	1	1	1	1	1	1	1	1	1	1
Severe, prolonged and repeated seizures	2	2	2	2	2	2	2	2	2	2
Alertness and attention										
Normal for age	0	0	0	0	0	0	0	0	0	0
Moderate deficit	1	1	1	1	1	1	1	1	1	1
Severe deficit	2	2	2	2	2	2	2	2	2	2
Hyperexcitability										
No signs	0	0	0	0	0	0	0	0	0	0
Signs compatible with normal life	1	1	1	1	1	1	1	1	1	1
Uncontrollable	2	2	2	2	2	2	2	2	2	2

4

Motor Development Milestones in the First 2 Years of Life

	Months
Head control	Months
Present before 4 months	0
Acquired during 5th or 6th month	1
Acquired after 6 months or absent	2
Sitting position	Months
Acquired before 9 months	0
Acquired between the 10th and 12th month	1
Acquired after 12 months or absent	2
Walking independently	Months
Acquired before 18 months	0
Acquired between the 19th and 24th month	1
Acquired after 2 years or absent	2
Putting a cube into a cup (by imitation)	Months
Acquired before 10 months	0
Acquired between the 11th and 14th month	1
Acquired after 14 months or absent	2
Grasping a pellet (thumb-index pinch)	Months
Acquired before 12 months	0
Acquired between the 13th and 15th month	1
Acquired after 15 months or absent	2
Building a three-cube tower (by imitation)	Months
Acquired before 21 months	0
Acquired between the 22nd and 24th month	1
Acquired after 2 years or absent	2

Passive Muscle Tone (Choose column I, II, or III according to corrected age)

Lower Limbs			I (1st–3rd Month)			II (4th–6th Month)			III (7th–9th Month)		
			Angle	Norm	Score	Angle	Norm	Score	Angle	Norm	Score
Adductors		R		≥40	0		≥70	0		≥100	0
		+		≤30	I		≤60	I		80–90	I
		L		NR*	2		NR	2		≤70	2
										NR	2
Asymmetry		R>L			X			X			X
		R<L			X			X			X
Popliteal angle		R		≥80	0		≥90	0		≥110	0
				≤70	I		≤80	I		90–100	I
				NR	2		NR	2		≤80	2
										NR	2
		L		≥80	0		≥90	0		≥110	0
				≤70	I		≤80	I		90–100	I
				NR	2		NR	2		≤80	2
										NR	2
Dorsiflexion of the foot		R					≤ 80	0		≤ 80	0
							90–100	I		90–100	I
							≥ 110	2		≥ 110	2
SLOW angle		L					≤ 80	0		≤ 80	0
							90–100	I		90–100	I
							≥ 110	2		≥ 110	2
Dorsiflexion of the foot		R					Identical	0		Identical	0
							Phasic str.	I		Phasic str.	I
							Tonic str.	2		Tonic str.	2
RAPID angle		L					Identical	0		Identical	0
							Phasic str.	I		Phasic str.	I
							Tonic str.	2		Tonic str.	2

*NR : no resistance

Upper Limbs

			I	II	III
Candlestick posture	R + L	Absent	0	0	0
		Present/fixed	X	X	X
Hand	R	Finger movements present	0	0	0
		Constantly closed hand	I	2	2
		Inactive thumb	2	2	2
	L	Finger movements present	0	0	0
		Constantly closed hand	I	2	2
		Inactive thumb	2	2	2
Scarf sign	R	Position I	0	I	2
		Position 2	0	0	0
		Position 3	2	0	0
		No resistance	2	2	2
	L	Position I	0	I	2
		Position 2	0	0	0
		Position 3	2	0	0
		No resistance	2	2	2

Comparison of the R and L Sides of the Body: Asymmetry Even Within the Normal Range

	I	II	III
Asymmetry absent or not categorized	0	0	0
Right side more tonic	I	I	I
Left side more tonic	I	I	I

Body Axis

		I	II	III
Dorsal extension	Absent or minimal	0	0	0
	Moderate	0	0	0
	Excessive (opisthotonos)	2	2	2
Ventral flexion	Moderate	0	0	0
	Absent or minimal	I	I	I
	Unlimited	2	2	2
Comparison of curvatures	Flexion ≥ Extension	0	0	0
	Flexion < Extension	I	I	I
	Excessive flexion and extension (rag doll)	2	2	2

Diffuse Rigidity

	I	II	III
No rigidity	0	0	0
Similar to the resistance felt when bending a lead pipe (independent of angles)	2	2	2

7

Motor Activity

	I	II	III
Face			
Facial expressions			
Varied and symmetrical	0	0	0
Insufficient	I	I	I
Drooling			
Absent	0	0	0
Present	X	X	X
Facial paralysis			
Absent	0	0	0
Present Side of face: _____	2	2	2
Fasciculations of the tongue (peripheral, at rest)			
Absent	0	0	0
Present	2	2	2
Limbs			
Spontaneous movements (quantitative and qualitative)			
Coordinated and varied	0	0	0
Insufficient, uncoordinated, stereotyped	I	I	I
Barely present and/or very uncoordinated	2	2	2
Involuntary movements			
Absent	0	0	0
Present Describe: _____	2	2	2
Dystonia			
Absent	0	0	0
Present	2	2	2

Deep Tendon and Cutaneous Reflexes

		I		II		III	
		R	L	R	L	R	L
Bicipital reflex	Normal	0	0	0	0	0	0
	Very brisk	I	I	I	I	I	I
	+ clonus	2	2	2	2	2	2
	Absent	2	2	2	2	2	2
Patellar reflex (knee jerk)	Normal	0	0	0	0	0	0
	Very brisk	I	I	I	I	I	I
	+ clonus	2	2	2	2	2	2
	Absent	2	2	2	2	2	2
Cutaneous reflex	Flexion	0	0	0	0	0	0
	Extension	X	X	X	X	X	X

8

Primitive Reflexes

Primitive Reflexes		I	II	III
Sucking	Present	0	0	0
	Insufficient	I	I	I
	Absent or completely inadequate	2	2	2
Moro reflex	Present	0	x	2
	Absent	2*	x	0
Grasping reflex	Present	0	x	2
	Absent	2*	x	0
Automatic walking reflex	Present	0	x	2
	Absent	2*	x	0
Asymmetric tonic neck reflex (ATNR)	Present, evident	x	x	2
	Absent	x	x	0
R/L asymmetry (Indicate affected side)				

*These observations are given a score of 2 only if other signs of CNS depression are present.

Postural Reactions

Postural Reactions		I		II		III	
		R	L	R	L	R	L
Lateral propping reaction while seated	Present					0	0
	Incomplete/absent					X	X
Parachute reaction (forward)	Present					0	0
	Incomplete/absent					X	X

Qualitative Abnormalities in Gross Motor Function and Acquired Deformities

Qualitative Abnormalities		I	II	III
Holding head behind the axis	Abnormality absent	0	0	0
	Abnormality present	X	X	X
Poorly maintained head control due to fatigue	Abnormality absent	0	0	0
	Abnormality present	X	X	X
Sitting position	Abnormality absent			0
	Falls forward (global hypotonia)			X
	Falls backward (hypertonia of the extensor muscles)			I
Standing position	Adequate reaction to standing	0	0	0
	Excessive extension in standing (opisthotonos)	2	2	2
Lower limb deformities	Deformity absent	0	0	0
	Scissoring of the legs	2	2	2

9

Passive Muscle Tone (Choose column IV, V, or VI according to corrected age)

Lower Limbs			IV (10th– 12th Month)			V (13th–18th Month)			VI (19th– 24th Month)		
			Angle	Norm	Score	Angle	Norm	Score	Angle	Norm	Score
Adductors		R		≥ 110	0		≥ 110	0		≥ 110	0
		+		80–100	1		80–110	1		80–100	1
		L		≤70	2		≤ 70	2		≤ 70	2
				NR*	X		NR	X		NR	2
Asymmetry		R>L			X			X			X
		R<L			X			X			X
Popliteal angle		R		≥ 110	0		≥ 110	0		≥ 110	0
				90–100	1		90–100	1		90–100	1
				≤ 80	2		≤ 80	2		≤ 80	2
				NR	X		NR	X		NR	2
		L		≥ 110	0		≥ 110	0		≥ 110	0
				90–100	1		90–100	1		90–100	1
				≤ 80	2		≤ 80	2		≤ 80	2
				NR	X		NR	X		NR	2
Dorsiflexion of the foot		R		≤ 80	0		≤ 80	0		≤ 80	0
				90–100	1		90–100	1		90–100	1
				≥ 110	2		≥ 110	2		≥ 110	2
SLOW angle		L		≤ 80	0		≤ 80	0		≤ 80	
				90–100	1		90–100	1		90–100	1
				≥ 110	2		≥ 110	2		≥ 110	2
Dorsiflexion of the foot		R		Identical	0		Identical	0		Identical	0
				Phasic str.	1		Phasic str.	1		Phasic str.	1
				Tonic str.	2		Tonic str.	2		Tonic str.	2
RAPID angle		L		Identical	0		Identical	0		Identical	0
				Phasic str.	1		Phasic str.	1		Phasic str.	1
				Tonic str.	2		Tonic str.	2		Tonic str.	2

*NR: no resistance

Upper Limbs			IV	V	VI
Candlestick posture	R + L	Absent	0	0	0
		Present/fixed	X	X	X
Hand	R	Finger movements present	0	0	0
		Constantly closed hand	2	2	2
		Inactive thumb	2	2	2
	L	Finger movements present	0	0	0
		Constantly closed hand	2	2	2
		Inactive thumb	2	2	2
Scarf sign	R	Position 2 or 3	0	0	0
		Position 1	2	2	2
		No resistance	X	X	2
	L	Position 2 or 3	0	0	0
		Position 1	2	2	2
		No resistance	X	X	2

Comparison of the R and L Sides of the Body: Asymmetry Even Within the Normal Range	IV	V	VI
Asymmetry absent or not categorized	0	0	0
Right side more tonic	1	1	1
Left side more tonic	1	1	1

Body Axis		IV	V	VI
Dorsal extension	Absent or minimal	0	0	0
	Moderate	0	0	0
	Excessive (opisthotonos)	2	2	2
Ventral flexion	Moderate	0	0	0
	Absent or minimal	0	0	0
	Unlimited	2	2	2
Comparison of curvatures	Flexion ≥ Extension	0	0	0
	Flexion < Extension	1	1	1
	Excessive flexion and extension (rag doll)	2	2	2

Diffuse Rigidity	IV	V	VI
No rigidity	0	0	0
Similar to the resistance felt when bending a lead pipe (independent of angles)	2	2	2

Motor Activity	IV	V	VI
Face			
Facial expressions			
Varied and symmetrical	0	0	0
Insufficient	I	I	I
Drooling			
Absent	0	0	0
Present	X	I	I
Facial paralysis			
Absent	0	0	0
Present Side of face: _____	2	2	2
Fasciculations of the tongue (peripheral, at rest)			
Absent	0	0	0
Present	2	2	2
Limbs			
Spontaneous movements (quantitative and qualitative)			
Coordinated and varied	0	0	0
Insufficient, uncoordinated, stereotyped	I	I	I
Barely present and/or very uncoordinated	2	2	2
Involuntary movements			
Absent	0	0	0
Present Describe: _____	2	2	2
Dystonia			
Absent	0	0	0
Present	2	2	2

Deep Tendon and Cutaneous Reflexes		IV		V		VI	
		R	L	R	L	R	L
Bicipital reflex	Normal	0	0	0	0	0	0
	Very brisk	I	I	I	I	I	I
	+ clonus	2	2	2	2	2	2
	Absent	2	2	2	2	2	2
Patellar reflex (knee jerk)	Normal	0	0	0	0	0	0
	Very brisk	I	I	I	I	I	I
	+ clonus	2	2	2	2	2	2
	Absent	2	2	2	2	2	2
Cutaneous reflex	Flexion	0	0	0	0	0	0
	Extension	X	X	2	2	2	2

Primitive Reflexes

Primitive Reflexes		IV	V	VI
Asymmetric tonic neck reflex (ATNR)	Absent	0	0	0
	Present, evident	2	2	2

Postural Reactions

Postural Reactions		IV		V		VI	
		R	L	R	L	R	L
Lateral propping reaction while seated	Present	0	0	0	0	0	0
	Incomplete	1	1	1	1	1	1
	Absent	2	2	2	2	2	2
Parachute reaction (forward)	Present	0	0	0	0	0	0
	Incomplete	1	1	1	1	1	1
	Absent	1	1	1	1	1	1

Qualitative Abnormalities in Gross Motor Function and Acquired Deformities

Qualitative Abnormalities in Gross Motor Function and Acquired Deformities		IV	V	VI
Holding head behind the axis	Abnormality absent	0	0	0
	Abnormality present	X	X	X
Poorly maintained head control due to fatigue	Abnormality absent	0	0	0
	Abnormality present	X	X	X
Sitting position	Abnormality absent	0	0	0
	Falls forward (global hypotonia)	1	2	2
	Falls backward (hypertonia of the extensor muscles)	1	2	2
Standing position	Normal reaction to standing	0	0	0
	Excessive extension in standing (opisthotonos)	2	2	2
Lower limb deformities	Deformity absent	0	0	0
	Scissoring of the legs	2	2	2

13

Passive Muscle Tone (Choose column VII at 2 years corrected and column V, VIII, IX, or X according to chronological age)

Lower Limbs			VII (3rd Year)		VIII (4th Year)		IX (5th Year)		X (6th Year)	
		Norm	Angle	Score	Angle	Score	Angle	Score	Angle	Score
Adductors	R + L	≥100 40–90 ≤30 NR*		0 1 2 2		0 1 2 2		0 1 2 2		0 1 2 2
Asymmetry	R>L			X		X		X		X
	R<L			X		X		X		X
Popliteal angle	R	120–160 100–110 ≤90 ≥160 NR		0 1 2 1 2		0 1 2 1 2		0 1 2 1 2		0 1 2 1 2
	L	120–160 100–110 ≤90 ≥160 NR		0 1 2 1 2		0 1 2 1 2		0 1 2 1 2		0 1 2 1 2
Dorsiflexion of the foot	R	≤ 80 90–100 ≥ 110		0 1 2		0 1 2		0 1 2		0 1 2
SLOW angle	L	≤ 80 90–100 ≥ 110		0 1 2		0 1 2		0 1 2		0 1 2
Dorsiflexion of the foot	R	Identical Phasic str. Tonic str.		0 1 2		0 1 2		0 1 2		0 1 2
RAPID angle	L	Identical Phasic str. Tonic str.		0 1 2		0 1 2		0 1 2		0 1 2

* NR: no resistance

14

Upper Limbs

			VII	VIII	IX	X
Candlestick posture	R+L	Absent	0	0	0	0
		Present/fixed	X	X	X	X
Hand	R	Finger movements present	0	0	0	0
		Constantly closed hand	2	2	2	2
		Inactive thumb	2	2	2	2
	L	Finger movements present	0	0	0	0
		Constantly closed hand	2	2	2	2
		Inactive thumb	2	2	2	2
Scarf sign	R	Position 2 or 3	0	0	0	0
		Position 1	1	1	1	1
		No resistance	2	2	2	2
	L	Position 2 or 3	0	0	0	0
		Position 1	1	1	1	1
		No resistance	2	2	2	2

Comparison of the R and L Sides of the Body: Asymmetry Even Within the Normal Range

	VII	VIII	IX	X
Asymmetry absent or not categorized	0	0	0	0
Right side more tonic	1	1	1	1
Left side more tonic	1	1	1	1

Body Axis

		VII	VIII	IX	X
Dorsal extension	Absent or minimal	0	0	0	0
	Moderate	0	0	0	0
	Excessive (opisthotonos)	2	2	2	2
Ventral flexion	Moderate	0	0	0	0
	Absent or minimal	0	0	0	0
	Unlimited	2	2	2	2
Comparison of curvatures	Flexion ≥ Extension	0	0	0	0
	Flexion < Extension	1	1	1	1
	Excessive flexion and extension (rag doll)	2	2	2	2

Diffuse Rigidity

	VII	VIII	IX	X
No rigidity	0	0	0	0
Similar to the resistance felt when bending a lead pipe (independent of angles)	2	2	2	2

15

Motor Activity	3rd–6th Year			
	VII	VIII	IX	X
Face				
Facial Expressions				
Varied and symmetrical	0	0	0	0
Insufficient	I	I	I	I
Drooling				
Absent	0	0	0	0
Present	2	2	2	2
Facial paralysis				
Absent	0	0	0	0
Present Side of face: _____	2	2	2	2
Fasciculations of the tongue (peripheral, at rest)				
Absent	0	0	0	0
Present	2	2	2	2
Limbs				
Spontaneous movements (quantitative and qualitative)				
Coordinated and varied	0	0	0	0
Insufficient, uncoordinated, stereotyped	I	I	I	I
Barely present and/or very uncoordinated	2	2	2	2
Involuntary movements				
Absent	0	0	0	0
Present Describe: _____	2	2	2	2
Dystonia				
Absent	0	0	0	0
Present	2	2	2	2

Deep Tendon and Cutaneous Reflexes		VII		VIII		IX		X	
		R	L	R	L	R	L	R	L
Bicipital reflex	Normal	0	0	0	0	0	0	0	0
	Very brisk	I	I	I	I	I	I	I	I
	+ clonus	2	2	2	2	2	2	2	2
	Absent	2	2	2	2	2	2	2	2
Patellar reflex (knee jerk)	Normal	0	0	0	0	0	0	0	0
	Very brisk	I	I	I	I	I	I	I	I
	+ clonus	2	2	2	2	2	2	2	2
	Absent	2	2	2	2	2	2	2	2
Cutaneous reflex	Flexion	0	0	0	0	0	0	0	0
	Extension	2	2	2	2	2	2	2	2

Primitive Reflexes		VII	VIII	IX	X
Asymmetric tonic neck reflex (ATNR)	Absent	0	0	0	0
	Present (elicited)			I	I
	Present evident	2	2	2	2

16

Postural Reactions		VII		VIII		IX		X	
		R	L	R	L	R	L	R	L
Lateral propping reaction while seated	Present	0	0	0	0	0	0	0	0
	Incomplete	2	2	2	2	2	2	2	2
	Absent	2	2	2	2	2	2	2	2
Parachute reaction (forward)	Present	0	0	0	0	0	0	0	0
	Incomplete	2	2	2	2	2	2	2	2
	Absent	2	2	2	2	2	2	2	2

Qualitative Abnormalities in Gross Motor Function and Acquired Deformities		VII	VIII	IX	X
Holding head behind the axis	Abnormality absent	0	0	0	0
	Abnormality present	2	2	2	2
Poorly maintained head control due to fatigue	Abnormality absent	0	0	0	0
	Abnormality present	2	2	2	2
Sitting position	Abnormality absent	0	0	0	0
	Falls forward (global hypotonia)	2	2	2	2
	Falls backward (hypertonia of the extensor muscles)	2	2	2	2
Poorly maintained sitting position due to fatigue	Abnormality absent	0	0	0	0
	Abnormality present	2	2	2	2
Acquired deformities	No deformities	0	0	0	0
	Scoliosis	I	I	I	I
	Kyphosis	I	I	I	I
Standing position	Normal reaction to standing	0	0	0	0
	Excessive extension in standing (opisthotonos)	2	2	2	2
Lower limb deformities	None	0	0	0	0
	Scissoring of the legs	2	2	2	2
	Permanent flexion of the hip	X	X	X	X
	Permanent flexion of the knee	X	X	X	X
	Equine deformity of the foot	X	X	X	X
	Dislocation of the hip	X	X	X	X
	Other Specify: _____	X	X	X	X
Gait	No abnormalities	0	0	0	0
	Spastic gait	X	X	X	X
	Ataxic gait	X	X	X	X
	Hemiplegic gait	X	X	X	X
	Walks with assistance	X	X	X	X

17

SUMMARY PROFILE AT 2 YEARS (CORRECTED AGE)
AND ANNUAL PROFILES UP TO 6 YEARS

Motor Function	2–3 Years	3–4 Years	4–5 Years	5–6 Years
No neuromotor signs				
Neuromotor signs, isolated or + cranial signs				
Confirmed CP (Clearly indicate type below)				
Topographical subtype				
Symptomatic subtype				
Walks unassisted				
Walks a short distance with assistance				
Unable to walk				

Deficits Other Than Neuromotor

Cognitive	Moderate				
	Severe				
Visual	Moderate				
	Severe				
Hearing	Moderate				
	Severe				
Epilepsy	Well controlled				
	Severe				
Behavioral problems	Moderate				
	Severe				

Problems Other Than Neurological

Growth				
Respiratory				
Digestive				
Retinopathy				
Other				

Socio-familial Conditions

Favorable				
Unfavorable				
Very unfavorable				

18

References

1. Amiel-Tison C, Stewart A. *The Newborn Infant: One Brain for Life*. Paris: INSERM-Doin; 1994.
2. Amiel-Tison C. *L'infirmité motrice d'origine cérébrale*. Paris: Masson; 1997.
3. Thomas A, Saint-Anne Dargassies S. *Études neurologiques sur le nouveau-né et le jeune nourrisson*. Paris: Masson; 1952.
4. Saint-Anne Dargassies S. *Neurological Development in the Full-Term and Premature Neonate*. Amsterdam: Elsevier; 1977.
5. Amiel-Tison C. A method for neurologic evaluation within the first year of life. *Curr Probl Pediatr* 1976;7(1):1–50.
6. Amiel-Tison C, Grenier A. *Neurologic Evaluation of the Newborn and the Infant*. New York: Masson; 1983.
7. Amiel-Tison C, Grenier A. *Neurological Assessment during the First Year of Life*. Goldberg R, trans. New York: Oxford University Press; 1986.
8. Amiel-Tison C, Stewart A. Follow-up studies during the first five years of life: a pervasive assessment of neurological function. *Arch Dis Child* 1989;64: 496–502.
9. Amiel-Tison C. Correlations between hypoxic-ischemic events during fetal life and outcome. In: Arbeille P, Maulik D, Laurini R, eds. *Fetal Hypoxia*. London: Parthenon Press; 1999.
10. Amiel-Tison C. Cerebral damage in full-term newborns: aetiological factors, neonatal status and long-term follow-up. *Biol Neonate* 1969;14:234–250.
11. Amiel-Tison C, Dubé R, Garel M, Jecquier JC. Outcome at age 5 years of full term infants with transient neurologic abnormalities in the first year of life. In: Stern L, ed. *Intensive Care*. Vol IV. New York: Masson; 1983:247–257.
12. Stewart AL, Reynolds EOR, Hope PL, et al. Probability of neurodevelopmental disorders estimated from ultrasound appearance of brains of very preterm infants. *Dev Med Child Neurol* 1987;29:3–11.

13. Stewart AL, Hope PL, Hamilton PA, et al. Prediction in very preterm infants of satisfactory neurodevelopmental progress at 12 months. *Dev Med Child Neurol* 1988;30:53–63.

14. Costello AM de L, Hamilton PA, Baudin J, et al. Prediction of neurodevelopmental impairment at 4 years from brain ultrasound appearance in very preterm infants. *Dev Med Child Neurol* 1988;30:711–722.

15. Stewart AL, Costello AM de L, Hamilton PA, Baudin J, et al. Relation between neurodevelopmental status at one and four years in very preterm infants. *Dev Med Child Neurol* 1989;33:756–765.

16. Amiel-Tison C, Njiokiktjien C, Vaivre-Douret L, et al. Relation of early neuromotor and cranial signs with neuropsychological outcome at 4 years. *Brain Dev* 1996;18:280–286.

17. Grenier A, Contraires B, Hernandorena X, Sainz M. Examen neuromoteur complémentaire au cours des premières semaines de la vie. Son application chez les nouveau-nés à risque. In: *Encyclopédie Médico-Chirurgicale*. 4090 A15-9. Paris: SGIM Les Martres-de-Veyre; 1988:1–10.

18. Grenier A, Hernandorena X, Sainz M, et al. Examen neuromoteur complémentaire des nourrissons à risque de séquelles. Pourquoi ? Comment ? *Arch Pédiatr* 1995;2:1007–1012.

19. Gosselin J. *Certains aspects métrologiques de l'examen neuromoteur complémentaire* [doctoral thesis]. Montreal: Université de Montréal; 1993.

20. Hoon AH, Pulsifer MB, Gopalan R, et al. Clinical adaptive test/clinical linguistic auditory milestone scale in early cognitive assessment. *J Pediatr* 1993;123:51–58.

21. Baron-Cohen S, Cox A, Baird G, et al. Psychological markers in the detection of autism in infancy in a large population. *Br J Psychiatry* 1998;168:58–163.

22. Rapin I, ed. Preschool children with inadequate communication: developmental language disorder, autism, low IQ. *Clin Dev Med* 1996;139 (special issue).

23. Child Growth Foundation. *Growth Charts: United Kingdom Cross-sectional Reference Data—1995/1*. London: Author; 1995.

24. Fenichel GM. Disorders of cranial volume and shape. In: *Clinical Pediatric Neurology: A Signs and Symptoms Approach*. 2nd ed. Philadelphia: Saunders; 1993:361–378.

Index